Healthy Perspectives

Healthy Perspectives

Living a Heart-Healthy, Diabetic-Friendly Lifestyle

LoriAnn Mathews

iUniverse, Inc.
New York Bloomington Shanghai

Healthy Perspectives
Living a Heart-Healthy, Diabetic-Friendly Lifestyle

Copyright © 2008 by LoriAnn Mathews

All rights reserved. No part of this book may be used or reproduced by any means, graphic, electronic, or mechanical, including photocopying, recording, taping or by any information storage retrieval system without the written permission of the publisher except in the case of brief quotations embodied in critical articles and reviews.

iUniverse books may be ordered through booksellers or by contacting:

iUniverse
1663 Liberty Drive
Bloomington, IN 47403
www.iuniverse.com
1-800-Authors (1-800-288-4677)

Because of the dynamic nature of the Internet, any Web addresses or links contained in this book may have changed since publication and may no longer be valid.

The views expressed in this work are solely those of the author and do not necessarily reflect the views of the publisher, and the publisher hereby disclaims any responsibility for them.

ISBN: 978-0-595-39745-7 (pbk)
ISBN: 978-0-595-84152-3 (ebk)

Printed in the United States of America

Contents

Introduction vii
CHAPTER 1   Perspective on Eating. 1
CHAPTER 2   Perspective on Fats 5
CHAPTER 3   Perspective on Carbohydrates 10
CHAPTER 4   Perspective on Fiber. 14
CHAPTER 5   Perspective on Proteins 16
CHAPTER 6   Instructions for Reading Labels 19
CHAPTER 7   Specific Ingredients 21
CHAPTER 8   Making it Work. 29
CHAPTER 9   Recipes 31
CHAPTER 10   Appetizers and Munchies. 32
CHAPTER 11   Soups. 52
CHAPTER 12   Salads 71
CHAPTER 13   Breads 116
CHAPTER 14   Main Course 142
CHAPTER 15   Vegetables 197
CHAPTER 16   Desserts 247
Index. 289

Introduction

After my husband's last physical he was diagnosed with heart disease and he was told he is also borderline diabetic. Our family doctor immediately referred us to a cardiologist, the first step was an angiogram to verify the potential clots. As I watched the blood flowing (or better yet not flowing) through my husbands heart on a monitor I realized that we had to change our lifestyle or we would be back in the hospital doing this again and maybe we wouldn't be as lucky next time, this time we found out through a physical, next time it could be a heart attack. Perry had four stents placed in the arteries around his heart and was told to change his diet and exercise to reduce the risk of on-going problems. The cardiologist was clear we had to change.

I also knew I was right on the edge of Type II Diabetes because I had been diagnosed with Poly Cystic Ovarian Disease years earlier and I have been showing signs of Insulin Resistance and gaining weight.

The sudden onset of these problems was just the wake up call we needed to change our lives. We changed everything!

Our lifestyle had to change completely or neither of us would be around to raise our youngest daughter. Years of study and research during college started to pay off personally, my degree is in family health. I thought I had learned what I needed to help my family live a healthy lifestyle, but I had not done a good job implementing it at all. I was also frustrated when I couldn't find complete information.

I could find recipes that were heart friendly (low in fat) or I could find recipes that were for a diabetic (low in carbohydrates), but I couldn't find anything that really fit the kind of lifestyle that would work. We had to be able to eat both healthy low fat meals that were made with healthy complex carbohydrates rather than with simple carbohydrates.

We meet with the dietician, who focused primarily on the diabetic issues. I was shocked to hear her advice was related to portion control rather than changing the foods we ate. Rather than flat out saying quit eating this and avoid that, she told us to eat smaller portions and to help control the diabetes. To me this felt like only part of the solution. I struggled with this and asked her why, she said, "We teach people what we think they will change not what they should change. A little improvement is better than none at all." She didn't seem interested in going outside of the set plan she had prepared, but I felt like we were capable of making more change, so I continued my research. I knew we could eat right and not starve. I decided I would find out what we should really be eating, what kind of foods we should completely avoid and figure our how to make it taste good.

My husband's heart doctor wanted him to reduce his saturated fat intake as much as possible and some how get his cholesterol down from 449 (bad cholesterol, LDL were 364 and the good cholesterol, HDL were 37) the doctor wanted his total cholesterol below 200, and he wanted the HDL above 40. For my husband a healthy diet alone would not solve the problem, his heritage gave him a big jump in cholesterol. So medication was an important component of his new lifestyle, but I also knew changing our lifestyle would improve his chances for success. I also didn't want him to also start on medication for diabetes.

So we started changing. What, when and how we ate. I knew for us to succeed the changes had to be simple enough to be able to do for the rest of our lives; this couldn't be a short-term change or a fad diet.

To be able to make drastic lifestyle changes they have to be easy and workable, particularly, if we expect to live this way for the rest of our life. There has to be some level of flexibility.

I started searching for information and recipes so we could eat healthy for both heart disease and reduce the risk for diabetes. I was frustrated when I couldn't find the recipes and information I needed to help my husband. My family needed recipes that would be both heart healthy and diabetic friendly, finding information and recipes for this combination was practically impossible. So over the past year I have researched and learned everything I can about healthy lifestyles for people with heart disease and diabetes and I have been creating recipes that are both heart healthy and diabetic friendly. This book contains information and recipes that are based on a whole foods concept. By using more healthy protein choices and whole grains, vegetables, and fruits to create meals that are both good tasting and healthy, we get back to less processed options.

I created this book for those who want to protect their heart health or those who have diabetes, but the advice is sound for anyone who wants to eat more healthfully. This book includes the methods and tools we learned and used to change our lifestyle, breaking things down to the simplest components. I know it works just by changing the way we eat my husband lost over 25 pounds and I lost 60.

First, look at what you eat. Why? Because like us you probably don't think you eat so badly. I thought we were like any other average family eating 3 meals a day with snacks sometimes we eat out, but generally eating healthy foods, I thought, but the silent offenders were killing us.

Those silent offenders are foods that are so common place that we don't even consider them a risk factor. We generally say white sugar is bad for us, but what about white flour, white rice, potatoes, high fructose corn syrup, hydrogenated oils, and saturated fats found in beef, pork and dairy products.

Can a diet that does not include common favorites like white sugar, potatoes and steak be any good? It's a tough question, but as you start to make changes daily and begin eating right you find out you can do it. You find the ability to adjust and you begin feeling better and having more energy.

After talking with the dietician and the doctor I realized they are just hoping to see some change in lifestyle, but they don't expect people to really change enough to keep themselves healthy without further medical treatment. Therefore, I'm not going to limit my discussion to what you might do, I'm going to discuss what I have found through extensive research and continued discussions with the doctor you can do to live a more healthy lifestyle. I'm sharing this information to reduce your frustration in searching for help, read it and then you can adapt the recommendations to fit your own family's lifestyle.

Let's start simple and then build on that.

Chapter 1
Perspective on Eating

Eating is a natural part of your survival that you can enjoy and not stress over. Because of serious health issues such as obesity and peer pressure, eating can become negative stress.

When we view eating food as stressful then eating right, losing weight and feeling good is even harder, almost impossible to accomplish If you're thinking to much about not "cheating," or what "I can't have", they become the major focus. It's like telling yourself not to think about purple elephants with pink polka dots, now don't you think about those purple elephants with pink polka dots. What are you thinking about?

Allow food to become your friend and ally. Food provides you with energy, nutrients, and pleasure. Don't spoil it by worrying about every little bite or calorie. Healthy eating can and should be a way to reduce stress in your life.

Learn to think about food as a gift and a valued friend. I know it sounds new age, but your mind has amazing control over what happens with your entire body, you need to learn to think healthy, and you will become healthy.

Right now, lets do this simple exercise.

Write down what your life will look like when you are healthy, be very descriptive, draw a picture if it will help. Include how you will feel, the activities you will do, are your muscles defined, and strong, what kind of stamina do you have, can you walk, jog or run? Are you able to do what you want, not what you can, considering your current physical limitations?

Remember a how your body felt when it was healthy regardless of what the scale may have said. Healthy isn't being a 105 pound, model with anorexia. It's being at a weight that allows you do be active and productive without limitations based on stamina.

Healthy is simple, you feel good and your body is able to do what you want and need and you are happy with it. Draw a reasonable picture, the focus is on health not appearance. One of the most important parts of my personal picture is being able to play with my 2 year old and not feel old (hey I'm 43 it wasn't any fun at 250 lbs.) Now I play more, laugh more and want her to be able to play and laugh more no matter how old she is.

Being healthy is a mental picture and getting to it takes the same kind of positive images and thoughts as succeeding in any avenue of life, business, sports, and/or family.

So visualize yourself healthy and strong and look at the picture over and over each day, implant health in your mind.

Repeat daily "I am healthy, I enjoy eating healthy foods that give me energy and my body is able to do what I want when I want."

Now to succeed, look at healthy perspectives as just that, a healthy way to look at issues. Apply what you feel good about and absorb the rest as knowledge. It will give you the ability to make more informed decisions about how to eat more healthy meals.

First, "Eat what you want once a month!"

If you thought you had had to give up your favorite foods forever to accomplish this, it probably would never work. You are not giving up any food forever. My husband's heart doctor advised us to do our best most of the time, but one meal a month we can eat whatever we want. You also have your Birthday, Thanksgiving and Christmas. These are considered special days when you don't worry about eating right, but be sure to get back on track the very next day.

There are also times when there is no option for food that fits within the plan. You may be at a conference; dinner at your parents, or in-laws, or some other special occasion. Do the best you can, but be careful not to offend those you care about learn to share with others how you have changed. Through your changes you may be a positive influence on them.

For example, due to health reasons, both my parents are now eating healthier and have made similar changes to ours. It has been an easier adjustment for them, because we shared our experiences.

Also, when you do slip, (and you will) don't think it's the end of the world, or the end of your new lifestyle changes. Don't give up. Just move forward and eat healthy the next meal.

Remember you're not giving it up any food forever; you just have to wait a few days for your free meal for the month and you can eat whatever you want.

Don't Count Calories

I preach a no calorie counting approach intentionally. It has to do with the mind set and worrying thing; by counting calories you focus only on the negative.

Worrying about each individual calorie makes it hard to eat healthy without the stress.

The dietician hit this one right on the nail, she taught us to eat portions instead of counting calories. Because even when you're eating the right kinds of foods eating too much of them will not lead to the healthy lifestyle. Count daily portions and you will succeed. Not eating too much even of a good thing is important, so follow the simple guidelines below to succeed.

Each day eat 7-9 portions of carbohydrates; 3-4 portions of protein; and a minimum of 5-8 servings of vegetables; minimize fats, especially animal based saturated fats.

A portion/serving of carbohydrates is about the same size as your fist or about 15 grams. Reading labels on foods will help you keep this simple. Generally you can eat 6-16 baked corn chips per serving. One slice of whole wheat bread is a portion. Fresh fruits and starchy vegetables are simple when you use the size of your fist.

A portion/serving of protein is easy to eyeball, it's the size of a deck of cards or the palm of your hand or about 4-5 ounces. We tend to eat larger portions than we need. Half a chicken breast is one portion. ½ cup of cottage cheese is a portion. If you eat more than a portion, count it as two.

Eat as many non-starchy vegetables, like broccoli, green beans, lettuce etc. as you like. Eat salads; fresh vegetables relish trays (with healthy dips recipes to follow). Vegetable soup is another great option.

Now how do you minimize fats? Avoid adding butter/oils for flavor; instead use spices, when cooking use spray oils and water. Do not deep fry or pan fry foods, instead oven fry or grill meats. Always read labels for hidden fats. We will discuss the importance of fat in our diet in the next chapter, because there are great fats like olive oil and omega 3 fatty acids found in salmon that our needs.

Eat often and eat good stuff.

The objective is not to starve yourself to good health, but to learn to eat right.

I promise you will not be hungry when you eat this way, in fact to really be healthy; you should be eating 5-6 small meals a day. The traditional 3 large meals a day sends the wrong signals to the brain. You are telling your body it has to wait to eat, so hold on to the energy I give you now (the body stores energy as fat). If we do not plan our meals, we tend to snack on whatever we can get our hands on throughout the day. Skipping meals will cause your body to store fat. When the body thinks you are going through a famine and therefore feeding it less it will start to hold on to everything. If you give the body what it needs it will let go of what it does not.

Eating often is important, but you don't need to eat a lot.

Starvation diets absolutely don't work, and skipping meals is the equivalent to starvation. The body knows storing fat is the most efficient energy source for survival; so it will burn lean muscle mass and convert what you eat into fat.

So what is considered a meal? Portions are important, not that you need to be weighing your food and measuring every serving, learning to eyeball saves you time and decreases the stress associated with eating.

Generally speaking a meal consists of a serving of protein, carbohydrate and vegetables. An evening snack may be a bowl of popcorn (no butter); a morning snack maybe an orange.

As we discuss foods and eating we are really talking about energy, that's what food really is. Food is digested by the body and converted into energy.

The greatest energy source is fats. They are easy to store, your body is able to convert them to energy easily, and gram for gram it provides the greatest amount of energy.

Proteins provide sustained energy. Your body works harder to break the proteins down, and therefore it provides energy over a longer period of time.

Carbohydrates provide quick energy. The body is able to utilize carbohydrates extremely fast. They also burn fast so the energy isn't lasting. The 2 types of carbohydrates are simple and complex.

A simple carbohydrate is digested and absorbed into the blood stream immediately, causing a spike in blood sugar levels. These spikes cause an immediate release of insulin. When your body has these spikes in blood sugar it begins to store the energy (converts it to fat). Complex carbohydrates take longer to digest and do not cause the same spikes in blood sugar levels.

Learning to provide the body with enough energy, and not too much, is the challenge we face. Understanding each of these energy sources helps us to better understand how to become friends with our bodies and the foods we eat.

Giving our bodies the right stuff, at the right time, is half the trick. The other half is ensuring the body has an opportunity to burn energy at an efficient rate. Our job is to create a balance between the in-coming and out-going energy.

Sounds complex? It is really very simple. Eat right and exercise. Eating smart and exercising smart, bring the best results.

Chapter 2
Perspective on Fats

Fat or oils provide energy as well as insulate, cushion and protect internal organs and help the body use carbohydrates and proteins more efficiently. No oil is completely made of just one type of fat; they all are a combination of the three fats (saturated, monounsaturated and polyunsaturated in different percentages.

For years, we've been told to consume as little fat as possible, but now, experts recognize that while too much fat is bad for you, some fat is a necessary part of our diet; fats are a source of essential nutrition. The trick is to consume the right kind and the right amount of fat or oil.

Did you know your body needs fat to burn fat? Choosing the right oils is essential for your health. These fats (polyunsaturated) slow down the absorption of carbohydrates, helping to control blood sugar. In addition, when we eat fat it causes the stomach to release CCK a hormone that tells the brain to stop eating. The following is a simple review of the major components of cholesterol and fats.

Cholesterol

The body will manufacture about 800-1500 mg. of cholesterol per day, contributing much more to total body cholesterol than the cholesterol we eat. Eating too much fat will encourage the body to make more cholesterol.

Excess cholesterol harms the body when it forms deposits on artery walls, leading to atherosclerosis and heart disease. Cholesterol can be further divided into HDLs and LDLs

Low-Density Lipoproteins (LDL)

Considered "bad" cholesterol. It is produced by the liver and circulates through the body, transporting fat to the muscles, heart, fat stores and other tissues.

High-Density Lipoproteins (HDL)

Considered "good" cholesterol. It is produced by the liver to carry cholesterol and phospholipids from the cells back to the liver for recycling and/or excretion. Because HDLs represent cholesterol removal from arteries and blood to the liver for breakdown and disposal, it is considered "good" cholesterol.

Fats to Avoid

Hydrogenated fats also known as Trans-fatty acids

Fat resulting from a process where hydrogen atoms are added to polyunsaturated or monounsaturated fats to protect against rancidity and make products more light and fluffy. This procedure effectively takes normally healthy oil and saturates it with hydrogen, making it quite simply deadly.

Trans-fatty acids increase "bad" LDL cholesterol and lower "good" HDL cholesterol. On the label you will see terms like partially hydrogenated oil or hydrogenated oil.

Hydrogenation increases the shelf life and flavor stability of foods containing these fats. Unlike other fats, the majority of trans fat is formed when food manufacturers turn liquid oils into solid fats like shortening and hard margarine.

Hydrogenated oil is created through a heating process. When fatty acids are overheated, it changes their molecular structure and they become mutated. The result is a trans-fatty acid, the most dangerous of all fats.

Think of trans-fatty acids as "sticky" fats that clog up the blood vessels, and slow down our metabolisms. Research has shown that hydrogenated fats are related to heart disease and circulatory problems.

Saturated fats—Usually solid at room temperature.

Animal fats that are solid at room temperature called saturated fats that will clog arteries causing heart disease; they play a major role in the production of cholesterol in the body. Primary sources of saturated fats are beef, pork and dairy products (butter).

There are 3 types of saturated fats, short, medium, and long chain (long are less healthy). Animal based saturated fats (long chain) can be detrimental to your health. These are generally found in all animals including fish and poultry, but the percentage of fat is much higher in beef, pork and dairy products.

On the other hand saturated fats found in tropical oils such as palm and coconut (medium chain) can have health benefits, when used in moderation and in conjunction with polyunsaturated fats.

Healthy Fats

Monounsaturated fats—Liquid at room temperature.

Monounsaturated fats include olive and canola oils. This type of fat tends to lower "bad" LDL cholesterol while leaving the "good" HDL cholesterol unchanged. The most widely used oils that are high in monounsaturated oils are olive oil, canola oil and peanut oil. Avocados, olives, and nuts are good sources of monounsaturated fats.

Polyunsaturated fats—Liquid at room temperature

Polyunsaturated fats include corn oil, safflower oil and sunflower oil. This type of fat tends to lower both "bad" LDL and "good" HDL cholesterol. Polyunsaturated fats, made up of omega-3 and omega-6 essential fatty acids are also considered relatively healthy.

Essential fatty acids

Linolenic Acid—The Omega-6 family and Omega-3 family. Common sources for these essential fatty acids are vegetable oils and meats.

Linolenic acid is a major component used by the brain and eyes, it is essential for growth and development. The body needs these fatty acids.

Fish, in particular, is abundant in both Omega-3 and Omega-6 fatty acids.

Oils high in omega-3 fatty acids are walnut oil, flaxseed oil and canola oil. Omega 3 fatty acids are also found in fresh deep-water fish: salmon, herring, tuna, sardines, mackerel, blue fish, and halibut. However, deep-frying or excessive heat can destroy the Omega-3 in these fish.

Omega-6 essential fatty acids are found in vegetable oils and salad dressings, safflower oil, sunflower oil, corn oil, and canola oil.

The body does not produce these Essential Fatty Acids so they must be supplied by the diet. They help our bodies synthesize other fatty acids, control the way cholesterol works, form the membranes of the cells in our bodies, and are a large part of the active tissue in our brains. Healthy fats actually help to clean out those sticky fats, promoting better health. They also speed up metabolism, helping to burn your food more efficiently, leading to weight loss.

On the market today are products such as Benecol, Smart Balance, etc. These are butter substitutes that will not cause health problems. They are acceptable when used in moderation; they contain the right fats and may help reduce cholesterol in your body. Do not eat regular margarine! It is hydrogenated fat or trans fat which is worse than saturated fats or butter.

Plant base Saturated Fats are also a healthy alternative to shortening and margarine for baking and cooking when used in moderation. These fats are found in coconut and palm oils.

Now that we understand a few oils or fats we can use to cook lets discuss how to use them for greater benefit and health.

When heating oil be careful not to heat burn it or cause it to smoke. When oil is heated past its smoke point it can cause it to have an off flavor, lose its nutritional value and turn the once healthy oil into trans fat. The process for creating trans fat is heat. So when cooking use oils that can handle the temperature, peanut oil for instance can be heated to high temperatures without smoking and changing its chemical compound. Oils that can take high temperatures make good all-purpose cooking oils. Choose from canola, sunflower and peanut for high-heat uses such as searing.

Using coconut oil in baked goods creates a flakier, light product, making it a good replacement for shortening and butter in baked goods.

Nuts are also a good source of healthy fats. Eating nuts can be very healthy and can help lower cholesterol, help reduce the risk of coronary heart disease, help to prevent Type II diabetes, and help prevent certain types of cancers as well as other benefits. They even help with weight control. Don't make the common mistake of avoiding nuts because they're too rich in fat and calories.

Almonds are one of the most concentrated, easy-to-eat sources of energy and nutrients. It's true that almonds, like other nuts, 170 calories per ounce and they contain 13 grams of fat per ounce. However, that fat is 87% monounsaturated fat, the kind that helps lower cholesterol and thus may protect you against heart disease

Almonds are high in vitamin E, which helps keep artery-clogging plaque at bay, thereby reducing your risk of high blood pressure, heart attacks, and stroke. Almonds are also an excellent source of calcium; they contain more of this mineral than any other nut, and are in fact one of the richest non-animal sources of calcium.

A few almonds also provide a hefty shot of protein. Almonds are 20% protein. An ounce of almonds contains about six grams of protein and the same amount of fiber; because fiber slows down the body's use of energy, almonds are a great source of slow-burning fuel.

Pecans contain heart healthy monounsaturated fat. Pecans are also good a source of vitamin E, magnesium, selenium, zinc, protein and fiber. Eating a small portion of pecans every day lowers the risk of fatal heart attacks and strokes. They also contain antioxidants that may prevent certain types of cancer; they may also help prevent obesity. Since pecans are high in fat, they have a high satiety value. People who eat them are less likely to get hungry quickly.

Walnuts are rich in alpha-linolenic acid, omega-3 fatty acid. They are also a good source of nutrients such as vitamin E and magnesium.

Peanuts are the most widely consumed 'nut' (actually a legume). Peanuts are a rich source of monounsaturated fatty acids, magnesium, copper, calcium, phosphorus, folic acid, fiber and vitamin E. The peanut contains more protein than any other legume or nut. You can get the same nutritional value from peanut butter as long as it does not contain added sugars.

Macadamia nuts are a high energy food. The natural oils in macadamias contain 80% monounsaturated fats. Macadamias are also a good source of protein, calcium, potassium and dietary fiber and are very low in sodium. Macadamias contain a higher level of monounsaturated fatty acids than any other commercial edible nut.

Chapter 3
Perspective on Carbohydrates

Food manufacturers have worked for years to create foods that are easy to serve and have a long shelf life. Although this may seem to be a benefit, in the end it may be the cause of several of the health problems we are facing today. Using simple carbohydrates that are inexpensive to mass produce and not considering the potential effect they may have on an individual's health continues to drive the market. The bottom line is profits are driving the industry, not what is best for you and your family.

By breaking down the carbohydrate so much our body does not need to do the work. The harder your body has to work to digest a carbohydrate the better. The problem is that most of the carbohydrates we are eating these days such as white bread, soda pop and potato chips have been processed and broken down so much that they turn to glucose (sugar) almost immediately in the blood stream. Our bodies are compensating by releasing insulin to process it. The body doesn't know what else to do with the sugar so it converts it to fat and stores it.

At best we just gain weight, but eventually the process may break down and our bodies become resistant to insulin and develop Type II diabetes.

The two types of carbohydrates are simple and complex.

Complex carbohydrates are primarily found in whole grains, cereals, nuts, beans, fruits and vegetables. These carbohydrates are absorbed by the body slowly and provide valuable nutrients to the body.

Simple carbohydrates or sugars are easily digested and turn to glucose in the blood stream fairly quickly. They are found in foods containing high fructose corn syrup, sugar, white flour, potatoes, white rice, and in the things we drink like juices, soda pop and alcohol. This list is very basic, learning to read labels is extremely important in this area. These ingredients can be found in almost every processed food you buy.

First, high fructose corn syrup, it is a manufacturers love this ingredient because it is made with corn which is readily available and cheap to process. It actually goes through a 12 step chemical process to be created, but it's still cheaper than cane or beet sugar and it has an unlimited shelf life. You can find it in almost every product you would expect to be sweet, but it is also hidden in products you would never suspect, like breads and cereals.

As a society we have become addicted to this over processed product. It's in soft drinks, juices, nutritional bars (suppose to be good for you), breads, cereals, condiments, salad dressings, and children's products like fruit snacks, cookies, candies, etc.

Now a little back ground on high fructose corn syrup. It is a highly concentrated sugar that is so broken down, your body doesn't have to do anything for it to become glucose in the blood stream. It sky rockets your blood sugar. Don't be fooled by the term fructose in the name, it is not a healthy sugar, far from it. It truly is leading the way to obesity and diabetes.

Reading labels is the only way to know if you are avoiding high fructose corn syrup. Because it is found in many foods you would not expect.

Second, sugar although not as bad as high fructose corn syrup, it is still a major contributor to health problems. Don't be fooled by the labeling, it may say "natural" or "organic", but that doesn't change anything, it's still sugar and it has been over processed for ease of use and storage; and the processing has made it easier for you body to absorb directly into the blood system and triggering insulin, adding to your risks of disease.

Eating whole foods and foods that have not been over processed allows our body to do the work. The body will absorb the food over time which prevents spikes in blood sugar and insulin release reducing the potential for fat storage.

Third, if you're eating white flour, potatoes and white rice you might as well be eating straight sugar. Your body treats them the same. That white bread my husband loved because he could roll it up in a ball and eat it, was turning to glucose immediately and raising his blood sugar with out any struggle and no need for the other functions of the body, just sugar.

To live a healthier lifestyle we need to eliminate or reduce our consumption of simple carbohydrates like high fructose corn syrup and decrease the amount of sugar, potatoes, white flour and rice, juices, soda pop and alcohol, in our daily life. This may seam a bit extreme, remember what the dietician said "we teach what we think they will change, not what they should." Making these kinds of changes is hard and takes a concentrated effort. It may not be easy to choose to brown rice over potatoes with dinner, or to choose whole wheat bread, my husband about went crazy when he started to eat his bologna on whole wheat bread (fat free bologna no less) but he's adjusted.

The value of change is obvious, when my husband was in the hospital after his heart surgery they served him a small bowl of white rice with his dinner, he ate it and two hours later tested his blood sugar. His blood sugar tested higher that night than any other time during testing. It shocked me how much one little bowl of rice could create such a high spike in blood sugar. White rice has been processed; all rice is brown before it goes through the milling process, which strips away the bran—and most of the nutrients—to make white rice.

Next, juices, this one was difficult for me. I love a glass of orange juice, but one small glass of orange juice is equal to the sugar of 3-4 oranges without any of the fiber or healthy carbohydrates. Because of the processing you get none of the fiber or other health benefits of the orange. Fruit is best eaten whole, leave the juice for your free meals. One small glass of fruit juice is equal to approximately 45 grams of carbohydrates or 3 portions.

Lastly, Alcohol is very rich in energy, packing 7 calories per gram. But like pure sugar or fat, the calories are void of nutrients. The more calories an individual consumes in alcohol, the less likely it is that they will eat enough food to obtain adequate nutrients.

To make matters worse, chronic alcohol use not only displaces calories from needed nutrients, but also interferes with the body's ability to metabolize nutrients, leading to damage of the liver, digestive system, and nearly every bodily organ.

Alcohol is very simply an extremely concentrated sugar. Yes, it does go through your liver to be processed but it has no nutritional value and raises your blood sugar levels extremely high. So simply put avoid alcohol.

So how much and what carbohydrates can you eat? Eating between 7 and 9 servings of complex carbohydrates a day will keep you on the track for health and wellness. Remember one serving is the size of your fist or approximately 15 grams. Avoid simple carbohydrates like sugar for these servings.

Let's talk about all the wonderful food just waiting for you to eat. Eat as many no starchy vegetables such as cucumbers, tomatoes, broccoli, lettuce, cabbage as you like (they don't count in your 7-9 servings). And eat a variety of them. Generally, they have a small amount of carbohydrates but not enough to worry about.

Eat salads with lots of fresh vegetable toppings, eat fresh, stir-fried and steamed vegetables, included are recipes for cooking vegetables.

Eat whole fruits; fruits that have very little effect on your blood sugar are cherries, plums peaches, and apricots. Generally fruits with pits have very little effect on your blood sugar, but most fruits are well within healthy ranges when eaten in moderation.

Eat breads in moderation but remember they have to be whole grain bread. If it doesn't say "whole" then it isn't. If it says enriched wheat flour that's just another way of saying white flour; if it says flour, white flour, enriched anything, then it is not whole wheat. It has to say "WHOLE WHEAT."

Whole grain pasta is a great source of carbohydrates, but read the labels and be sure they are whole wheat. If your dining out request whole wheat pasta. Remember 1 carbohydrate serving is the size of your fist, so you need to count it as 2-3 if you eat more.

I have found whole wheat, low fat tortilla shells that make great tacos. But check to be sure they are not made with hydrogenated fats. You can also find whole wheat crackers.

So how do you sweeten foods, if you can't eat sugar or high fructose corn syrup? Using less processed sweeteners in moderation is the key. These sweeteners include; honey, molasses, real maple syrup, barley malt, and evaporated cane juice. Remember these are to be used in small quantities.

The sweetness these sweeteners provide can be more intense and slightly different than sugar, so you need to learn to adjust recipes. The more you lighten up on the sweets, the less you will crave them (the ingredients section clearly explains each of these).

Focusing on eating primarily complex carbohydrates will help you keep your blood sugar levels from fluctuating. Fluctuations in blood sugar can cause health problems such as obesity and diabetes.

Everything we've discussed is designed to help you maintain stable blood sugar levels.

Chapter 4
Perspective on Fiber

Dietary Fiber is a carbohydrate that cannot be completely digested and is classified as either soluble or insoluble; both are important to a healthy diet.

Soluble fiber is found in nuts, vegetables, oats, oat bran, oatmeal, beans, peas, rice bran, barley, citrus fruits, strawberries and apple pulp, it has been proven to help reduce cholesterol while slowing digestion in the stomach keeping blood sugar levels consistent. Soluble fiber helps guide insulin into individual cells and out of the bloodstream. Eating just one-half cup of dried beans a day has been shown to significantly improve blood sugar control.

Insoluble fiber helps keep the digestive system moving and can be found in whole wheat, wheat bran and many vegetables such as broccoli, spinach, swiss chard, green peas and other dark green leafy vegetables dried peas and beans such as kidney beans, lima beans, black-eyed beans, chick peas and lentils.
It is easy to choose whole-grain foods at meals throughout the day. Simply do some of the following:

- Breakfast cereal with bran or a bowl of oatmeal is a good start.

- At lunch, choose whole wheat for your sandwich. All bread is not equal in fiber, so be sure to check the nutrition label.

- Brown rice and wild rice make great side dishes.

Dry beans and lentils are great sources of soluble fiber. They have lots of protein and may be selected as a meat replacement. Aim to include dry beans and legumes at least two to three times each week. All that fiber, along with plentiful complex carbohydrates, also makes legumes a great choice for anyone who wants steady, slow-burning energy. The best fiber choices include: black-eyed peas, kidney beans, chickpeas, lima beans, and black beans.

Try the following suggestions for easy ways to incorporate more beans into your diet

- Black beans and brown rice
- Add black beans or corn to salsa and chips
- Make tacos with fat-free refried beans.
- Add canned beans to vegetable soup.
- Eat the whole fruit or vegetable.
- Use raw spinach leaves in your salad.
- Add lots of carrots and other vegetables to the salad. Beets and chickpeas, raisins, sunflower seeds, and chopped apples
- Wash pieces of fruit each day so that they will be easy to grab for snacks and meal preparation.
- Keep carrot, celery and pepper strips ready to nibble.
- Add fresh spinach, tomatoes, sprouts, cucumbers, or peppers to you sandwich.

Chapter 5
Perspective on Proteins

Protein is a major part of the body—found primarily in muscle. We need protein for the growth and repair of tissues without it we could not survive. Your muscles, your organs, and your immune system are made up mostly of protein.

Your body uses the protein you eat to build up, maintain, and replace the tissues in your body and to make hemoglobin, the part of red blood cells that carries oxygen to every part of your body. The best sources of proteins are meat, poultry, fish, eggs, dairy products, nuts, seeds, and legumes.

During digestion, proteins are broken down into smaller units called amino acids. There are 20 different amino acids, which can be combined to make many different proteins. Our bodies can make proteins from amino acids, but we're unable to produce nine of the acids. These are known as essential amino acids and must be supplied by our diet.

When you eat foods that contain protein, the body breaks down the protein into amino acids. The amino acids then can be reused to make the proteins your body needs to maintain muscles, bones, blood, and body organs.

Only some foods are considered complete because they contain all the essential amino acids. These are milk and dairy products, eggs, fish, meat and poultry.

Most vegetable protein is considered incomplete because it lacks one or more of the essential amino acids.

For instance, you can't get all the amino acids you need from peanuts alone, but if you have peanuts or peanut butter on whole-grain bread it makes a complete protein. Likewise, red beans won't give you everything you need, but red beans and brown rice will do it.

The good news is that you don't have to eat all the essential amino acids in every meal. As long as you have a variety of protein sources throughout the day, your body will get what it needs from each meal.

Meats and Poultry

Remember beef and Pork are both extremely high in saturated fats and therefore should be avoided. So how do you get enough protein without eating beef or pork? Oh it's possible to get all the protein you need and more. You can still eat meat, but you can to choose to eat buffalo, turkey, chicken or elk instead of beef and pork. Buffalo is actually leaner than chicken and turkey and cooks and taste almost like beef. It does not have a gamy flavor or after taste. It is available through health food stores, local butchers and there are some resources on the internet. I use buffalo to make everything from hamburgers to chili and we have great steaks.

Elk is also available through the internet and is as lean as poultry. To prepare it, you need to marinade and spice more carefully because it does have a slight gamy flavor. I use it for tacos, chili and stews that will cook for a while with spices.

Turkey and chicken are both excellent sources of protein and are relatively low in saturated fats, provided you cook them without skins and you use only the white meat. The fats are stored in the skins and dark meat. Cooking the meat with the skin on allows the fat to soak into the meat, so you need to remove the skin.

Ground turkey is readily available and makes healthy meal preparation easy. But again read the labels, you may think you are buying lean ground turkey, but it may be a combination of white and dark meat and have as much fat as beef.

Fish is another excellent source of protein, although salmon is a high fat food, the fat is healthy fat and you should make an effort to eat deep, cold water fish twice a week. Other deep, cold water fish are halibut, tuna, orange roughy, herring and blue fish.

My favorite method for preparing fish is on my George Foreman Grill™. It is fast and it never seems to dry the fish out. I can prepare a full meal in less than a ½ hour.

I use my George Foreman™ grill for preparing chicken, fish and vegetables. It makes an extremely healthy option because most fat that was there is drained out and because it is cooking both sides at the same time it is fast. It is much more convenient than cooking on the grill outside.

You need to avoid shell fish, such as shrimp, lobster and crab. All of these types of fish are both high in fats and cholesterol.

Eggs

Although eggs are a great source of protein, the egg yolks are too high in saturated fats to be considered healthy. A great substitute is Egg Beaters, or other egg white only substitutes. Egg Beaters are made with egg whites and therefore have all the protein benefits and none of the fat. You can use them in all cooking. One quarter cup equals 1 whole egg. I generally use egg whites for baking. Also, egg white sandwiches make a great breakfast.

Beans and Legumes

Vegetarians have relied on legumes, dried beans and peas, as a nutritious source of non-animal protein. Like meat, beans are loaded with protein; unlike meat, they're not loaded with fat and calories.

Beans contain incomplete rather than complete protein. Therefore you need to combine beans with a starch such as brown rice or corn to provide the complementary protein.

Although beans and starches make a natural combination, you don't have to have them together in order to obtain complete protein; as long as you get two complementary proteins during the course of the day, you'll be fine.

Canned beans are just as nutritious as dried beans and will do just as much to help lower cholesterol. But be sure to rinse them well first; they are generally packed in high sodium liquid, to extend their shelf life.

Dairy Products

Dairy products are another good source of protein, but again because they are animal products they are high in saturated fats. Nonfat products are available.

Fat free products are available such as skim or nonfat milk; nonfat cottage cheese; Kraft™ makes a grated fat free mozzarella, cheddar cheese and sharp slices. These are the best tasting fat free cheeses we have found. Be careful with part skim mozzarella, it still contains a fair amount of saturated fats. You may be able to find reduced fat cheese, just be sure you are not getting more than about 5 grams of saturated fat per serving.

How Much Protein Is Enough?

Adults need approximately 3-4 portions of protein a day. You can look at a food label to find out how many protein grams are in a serving. But if you're eating a balanced diet, just monitor to ensure you're getting your portions; it is pretty easy to get enough protein.

Chapter 6
Instructions for Reading Labels

Start by reading every label in your pantry. Look for the following information on the label.

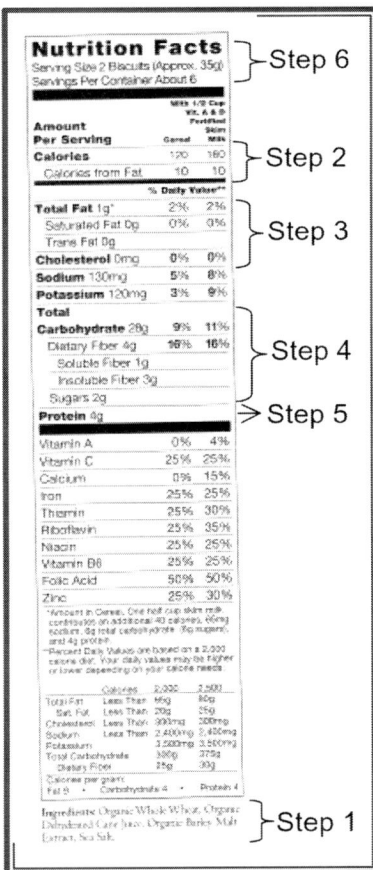

Step 1-read the ingredients list, confirm everything is good for you and you want to eat it. Your catsup has high fructose corn syrup. So read each ingredient. If it has a good balance of ingredients and does not have foods in the avoid or do not eat list then move forward.

Step 2—Look at how many calories are from fat. If more than 30% reconsider the item (unless the item is part of the fat group such as nuts, Benecol or oils).

Step 3—Now we start looking at Nutritional content. First look at the fat. We are looking for how much of each type of fat it has, if more than 30% of the fat is saturated; it is probably a food you should avoid. If it has any trans fat, then stay away from it.

Step 4—Now look at total carbohydrates, keep in mind each portion of carbohydrates is approximately 15 grams, so in this product, one serving is equal to 2 portions. Check how much comes from sugars. The more sugar the more quickly it will digest into the blood stream. So determine if you want to use your valued carbohydrates eating this product.

Step 5—Take a look at how many grams of protein. A portion of protein is 6-12 grams. You will get proteins from unexpected foods. There are 4 grams in this whole-wheat cereal.

Step 6—Pay close attention to serving sizes. You can eat too much of a good thing if you don't realize you're only suppose to eat 2 biscuits per serving.

Chapter 7
Specific Ingredients

The following is designed as an aid when shopping to help you find healthy food choices.

Grains and Flours

Bran—Coarse miller's bran is an excellent source of fiber, preventing many digestive and colon problems. It is rather bland and not easily detected when added to baked goods.

Cornmeal—Look for stone ground or water ground cornmeal. It is less processed and maintains more of its nutritional value.

Oats—Somehow oats survive the refining process with most of its nutrients intact. Oats are a good source of B vitamins, calcium, potassium and protein.

Popcorn Flour—This is one you have to make yourself. You make if from freshly popped corn. Do not add any salt or oil. It is best to use an air popper and use a food processor to grind it up and then sift it for best results.

It is light and airy and helps to lighten the weight of baked goods. Only add a little to breads and muffins. Because it is so light you have to use it with other flours.

Rice Flour—Made from brown rice, rice flour is a good source of iron, protein, minerals, and B vitamins. It is extremely low in sodium, so it is a good substitute for those who need a salt free diet.

Wheat Bran—Bran is the outer coating of the wheat berry. It is a good source of B vitamins, and minerals and an excellent source of fiber. Bran is an aid to the digestive system and has been shown to protect against gallbladder disease. It decreases the absorption of cholesterol and unfriendly fats.

Wheat Germ—The wheat germ is the heart or essence of life; wheat germ is rich in life giving nutrients that makes bread the staff of life.

Unless you are using whole-wheat flour, the germ has been removed. It has been removed from the processed food you can find on the shelves at the grocery store.

Wheat germ provides protein, the B vitamins, and minerals. Store wheat germ in the freezer and it will last longer.

Whole Wheat Flour—Ground from hard wheat and is high in gluten, which means the flour will absorb more liquid. Whole Wheat Pastry Flour is recommended for baking. Its finer texture is easier to substitute for white flour in most recipes. (Beware that wheat is one of the most common allergens, if this is the case then using Millet flour as a substitute works well).

Fats

Generally I cook with either Canola or Olive Oil; and Pam™ cooking spray.

Canola Oil—Good for general cooking and baking; it has no noticeable flavor and can be cooked at a medium high temperature.

Olive Oils—Extra Virgin Olive Oil has the most distinct flavor and you also need to use lower temperatures when cooking with it. Pure Olive Oil has no real flavor and can be used for cooking. Use both depending on what you are preparing.

When you purchase processed food, you can have peanut, sesame, safflower, sunflower, soy or corn oils, but remember nothing that says "hydrogenated".

Butters and Margarines are no longer an option. If you are choosing between butter and margarine at a restaurant then absolutely use butter. Margarine is generally made of trans fats and therefore the worst of the worst.

When baking replace butter, shortening, or margarine with coconut oil it will help maintain the consistency, without adding health risks.

But the latest products on the market to assist with decreasing cholesterol and providing flavor are butter substitutes that help reduce cholesterol. These products are labeled clearly. Benecol™ seems to have the best flavor, use it for buttering bread or when the flavor will be obvious. Cooking with Smart Balance™ gives you enough flavor and it is less expensive then Benecol.

Salad Dressings can be full of f fat and sugar Be careful to read labels carefully to ensure the type of fats and type of sweeteners are okay. Generally if the dressing is low fat then you better pay closer attention to the sugar content.

One salad dressing that is made of both the right kinds of fat and generally the right kind of sweeteners is "Brianna's™". Brianna's™ is made with either canola or olive oil and made with honey. Sometimes it is made with a small amount of sugar, but it never has high fructose corn syrup.

Just because it has the right kinds of fats and sweeteners, does not mean you can have unlimited amounts, again watch portions and use only enough to add the flavor.

Sweeteners

Do not use either white or brown sugar, they are both highly processed and refined and have no nutritional value. They are empty and easily metabolized. These sugars go directly to the blood stream and trigger an over production of insulin. The sugar you eat will be converted to fat and stored by the body. The following is a list of several sweeteners you can use in moderation.

Honey—Twice as sweet as sugar, so you only need half as much honey. It is absorbed into the blood stream slower and is less likely to cause the sugar spike. If your honey crystallizes don't worry. Just put it in warm water and you'll be able to use within minutes.

Clover honey has the mildest flavor and so it can be used in baked goods; your family will hardly notice the difference.

When converting recipes the general rule is to use only a ½ cup of honey for every cup of sugar called for in the recipe. Reduce the liquid or increase the flour to compensate for the extra liquid in honey. Usually you can add about ½ cup of flour for every cup of honey. Also, cook at a slightly lower temperature. Decrease your oven temperature by 25 degrees.

Maple Syrup—Made from the boiled sap of sugar maple trees maple syrup is a good sweetener used in moderation. Look for pure, 100% maple syrup. Most of the syrup on the shelves is actually just maple flavor corn syrup.

USDA Grade A maple syrup is the most popular grade for everyday use as a topping on pancakes, desserts, and other foods. USDA Grade B syrup is much darker and has a stronger flavor, which makes it more suitable for flavoring and cooking purposes. When baking with maple, use it just like you would honey, but remember you will get a distinct flavor from the syrup.

Molasses—Made from the juice of the sugar cane, molasses has been through minimal processes. It is high in calcium, potassium and iron. It is about half as sweet as sugar and has a distinct flavor. Use it in conjunction with honey for a more balanced taste.

Evaporated Cane Juice—Evaporated cane juice is a healthier alternative to refined sugar. While both sweeteners are made from sugar cane, evaporated cane juice does not undergo the same degree of processing that refined sugar does. Therefore, unlike refined sugar, it retains more of the nutrients found in sugar cane.

Evaporated cane juice can be used just like sugar for sweetening foods and beverages, as well as in cooking. But remember because it is a sugar you need to use it sparingly and rarely.

Sorghum Syrup—Made from 100% pure, natural juice extracted from sorghum cane. The juice is cleansed of impurities and concentrated by evaporation in open pans into clear, amber colored, mild flavored syrup. The syrup retains all of its natural sugars and other nutrients. When you see labels that say grain sweetened they are usually referring to Sorghram.

Eggs

I use Egg Beaters for breakfast and when preparing savory foods. Egg whites work well for baking. Avoid using the whole egg, because the yolk contains all the fat and cholesterol.

Cocoa

Unsweetened cocoa can be used in recipes, but use it sparingly because of the fat content. Cocoa is an excellent source of antioxidants and can be part of a healthy lifestyle.

Ingredients for Flavor

Can you imagine eating bland, flavorless food? I know I would never survive if I had to eat boring food. This section will discuss several flavor options that will enhance your pleasure experience with food with out increasing your risk for disease.

I use peppers, herbs and spices, and other ingredients to change and accent the foods I cook. Be willing to try different combinations when you cook and you will discover even more options than you will find in this guide. If your new combination works, great, if not youu learned something form the experiment.

Peppers

Peppers are wonderful. All different kinds are great. They add incredible flavor without adding carbohydrates or fats. Whether you like your food mild or spicy, you can create good flavor through peppers.

Each pepper has a slightly different flavor and intensity. Remember by removing the ribs and seeds you will reduce the heat of the pepper.

Sweet peppers are those that have very little bite to them or none at all,

Bell Peppers are delicious eaten fresh in green and pasta salads, and make a wonderful addition to spaghetti sauce. One of the most common bell pepper recipes, however, is Stuffed Bell Peppers.

Relleno Peppers have a very mild taste and are the traditional stuffing pepper, they are delicious stuffed, roasted or fried.

Anaheim chili peppers are good stuffing, grilling, roasting and pickling peppers. These are the mild green chilies you can find canned, but I prefer them fresh. I make my salsa with these.

Jalapenos are one of the hotter medium peppers, they are popular in Mexican cooking—fresh, pickled and dried. When smoke dried, jalapenos are known as chipotles.

Cayenne Peppers are very popular in Indian and Indo-Chinese cooking for curries and other hot dishes. It is also used frequently in Creole and Cajun dishes.

Serrano Peppers are an "all-purpose" hot pepper perfect for hot sauces, they add a wonderful flavor to guacamole and chili.

Habanero Peppers have a sweet, plum tomato-apple flavor under the heat. The sweetness of fruit often counterbalances the super heat of habanero peppers, try combining it with peaches or apricots to make tangy-sweet dish.

Thai Hot Peppers are popular in Asian cooking, especially stir-fry dishes. They are very hot with a heat that lingers.

No matter how you choose to use the peppers, they will add variety and flavor to your meals.

Spices and Herbs

Using fresh or dried herbs and spices will also add flavor. Review the following and be creative, use them slightly different than you have in the past and you will discover new and delicious meals. Don't be afraid to be untraditional, you can experiment with combinations.

Mint has a spicy sweet menthol flavor. Try it with tea, black beans, eggplant, lentils, and tomato-based dishes.

Rosemary has a piney flavor with hints of lemon. Try it with mushrooms, salmon, and beans.

Oregano classically used in tomatoes and pizza, try with either fish or summer squash.

Savory is a cross between thyme and mint. Its most often cooked with beans, especially bean soup, but use it also on grilled chicken.

Sage is somewhat bitter and has a musty-mint flavor. Try it with tomatoes, grilled tuna or other oily fish, and grilled poultry.

Thyme is one of the most basic herbs, having a pungent, minty, light lemon aroma with a hint of clove use it to flavor stocks and soups, and with all meats.

Basil is a cross between licorice and cloves. Basil is extremely versatile. Besides the obvious tomatoes, it goes especially well with poultry, fish, in salads and combined with all vegetables.

Parsley has a slightly peppery flavor. The flat leafed has the best flavor. Try it with chicken, eggs, fish, pasta, and vegetables.

Coriander or Cilantro, The leaves are sold as Cilantro; the seeds are sold as Coriander. This is a very pungent herb that people seem to love or hate. It is very popular in Mexican and Thai cuisine; it would be hard to have good salsa or guacamole without cilantro. Use cilantro also with chicken, fish, and vegetables. Try combining coriander with lentils or other dried beans. Add coriander to any dish that has ginger.

Cumin, on a worldwide basis, is the second most popular spice behind pepper. It is very compatible with hot chilies—you would recognize cumin's flavor in any prepared Chile dish. Try it also in bean soups, and with chicken.

Dill leaves are used as an herb; the seeds as a spice. Some people like dill's tang. The seeds are classically paired with cucumbers to make dill pickles. The leaves are most commonly used with salmon and other fish.

Bay Leaf is pungent and piney, and, unlike most fresh herbs, can be cooked for a long time in a sauce and can be used in stocks, soups, or stews. Try a little in grain dishes.

Chives have a mild onion flavor. Besides being a great garnish, they add a little zip to salads, especially in the vinaigrette. Use them where you would use onions, but add them at the last minute to get their full flavor.

Tarragon has a predominant licorice flavor. It is especially compatible with chicken and turkey as well as most vegetables. Throw some in a salad.

Mustard comes in either a powder form or as seeds. It is very hot; the temperature of prepared mustard is determined by dilution. Besides providing the base for the condiment, the powder can be added to vinaigrette. The seeds can be used in barbecue sauce.

Turmeric is a spice is valued mostly as a great dye—it turns anything yellow. It is used in curries, chicken or even bread.

Garlic is used as a savory seasoning for almost every type of meal. Aromatic and almost bitter when raw, garlic becomes delicate and sweet when cooked. Whenever possible you should use fresh garlic.

Black or White Pepper adds a mild spice to just about any food. This is a favorite at our house. Adding pepper livens up just about any dish. To make white pepper, the berries are allowed to ripen further, and then the black covering is stripped. White pepper has less heat than black pepper. It is usually used when black specks are undesirable.

Vanilla is an essential dessert spice, there is a substantial difference between real and artificial vanilla, and the real is worth the extra price. Vanilla can add mystery to fish dishes.

Cinnamon is the most common baking spice. Cinnamon is used in baked goods such as cookies, and desserts. Cinnamon is also used in savory chicken dishes from the Middle East.

Cloves are used whole to flavor stock, while ground cloves are found in baked goods. Cloves are also compatible with buffalo–throw some in the marinade.

Nutmeg can be used in barbecue sauces or try it on a variety of vegetables like spinach and carrots.

Allspice adds a touch of sweetness to desserts. Besides baking, it can be used on a surprising variety of foods such as meats, onions, squash and carrots.

Poppy seeds come in both blue and white varieties—the blue is sweeter and used in desserts while Indians prefer to use the white in their cooking. Add poppy seeds to salad dressings, especially if the dressing is to be used on fruit salads.

Ginger, especially grated freshly, has historically been used in Asia. Ginger is now widely used outside of baking. Try it on tomatoes, onions, or in chicken soup.

Using herbs and spices will provide variety, but be sure to use the right amounts. When using fresh herbs, use three times what you would for dried herbs. Gently wash them prior to use and add them towards the end of food preparation. The flavor is best when cooked less time.

Vinegar

Vinegar is a great way to flavor and tenderize. I use vinegar in marinades and dipping sauces. It adds a nice tangy flavor without adding

Balsamic Vinegar is distinctive Italian vinegar aged in wooden barrels for at least 10 years. To enjoy it at its best, don't heat balsamic vinegar, drizzled over grilled meats or toss with ripe fresh berries.

These vinegars have a sweet, pungent quality that works well to make a deglazing sauce or when used in salad dressings or to season slow-cooked meats and stews.

Cider Vinegar has a fruity apple flavor. Use cider vinegar to make a deglazing sauce for meats or in vinaigrette. Its mild flavor also makes it good vinegar to use for pickles.

Flavored Vinegars are made from wine vinegars (usually white wine) infused with fruits and/or fresh herbs. Use them to add a subtle herbal or fruit flavor to your salads, chicken, or fish.

Raspberry vinegar is one of the most flavorful fruit vinegars and tarragon vinegar is one of the best herb vinegars. It has a fabulous flavor for salads and fish.

Red Wine Vinegar has a bold flavor, combine it with mustard and shallots for bold flavored vinaigrette.

White Rice Vinegar has a pale, golden color and delicate flavor and extremely versatile. Use white rice vinegar for chicken, fish, and vegetables.

Sherry Vinegar is sweeter and more complex than ordinary wine vinegar. Sherry vinegar is aged for a minimum of 6 years in a network of barrels known as a solera. Sherry vinegar makes extraordinary vinaigrettes and can also be used to deglaze a roasting pan for chicken.

Others

Fruit Zest is great for flavoring in both baked goods and savory meat dishes.

Onions are great for flavoring. Yellow onions are full-flavored and are a reliable standby for cooking almost anything. Yellow onions turn a rich, dark brown when cooked and give French Onion Soup its tangy sweet flavor.

The red onion, with its wonderful color, is a good choice for fresh uses or in grilling and charbroiling.

White onions are the traditional onion used in classic Mexican cuisine. They have a golden color and sweet flavor when sautéed.

Remember the Do Not Eat List Consists of the Following Ingredients:

High Fructose Corn Syrup

Hydrogenated or Partially Hydrogenated Fats

White Sugar

White Flour

White Rice

Potatoes (except sweet potatoes)

Fruit Juices

Alcohol

Beef

Pork

Fat laden Dairy Products

Chapter 8
Making it Work

All of the information in this guide is to assist you in creating a lifestyle you can live with for the rest of your life. Making temporary changes will not work. As you go through the process of cleaning out your cupboards and start shopping for foods that are healthier for you and your family, keep in mind this is a process, not a final destination.

Life will continue to happen and you will run into roadblocks that will challenge your resolve to stay the course. When this happens take the time to remember why you started in the first place. Keep your goals of good health paramount in your decision making process. Study each of the Healthy Perspectives and take them to heart. Realize they are intended as a guide, not a restriction. We each have the ability to learn and apply new knowledge no matter how old or set in our ways we may be, but we have to choose to change.

The most satisfying realization for me through this entire project has been watching both my husband and my parents change. Even more satisfying than the changes I have made in my life. My family has been willing made drastic changes to improve their health and they have trusted me to study and find the correct information for them. They have applied the guidelines in Healthy Perspectives and they have lost weight, lowered their cholesterol, reduced their risks for diabetes, by balancing their blood sugar levels, and they have found more energy.

We are no longer stressed about our lifestyle and we are becoming healthier each day. That is my goal for you as well. That you will feel healthier, be more relaxed about eating and be able to accomplish your goals in life.

Next you will find several recipes that will help you apply the principles of Healthy Perspectives. They are all healthy and use only the best ingredients. Cooking with whole foods is slightly different than using processed foods, some may take a little more time to prepare, and they have a different flavor and constituency than you may be accustomed to, so be willing to try them anyway. Plan your days and meals so you have the needed time to cook your meals. Several of the recipes can be prepared in less than an hour, but some may take more time. Preparing things like brown rice the night before will speed up the process of preparing your meals.

Take the time each week to plan your menu and you will be able to prepare foods for more than one meal at a time. Prepare your lunch and snacks for the next day at night. Remember to plan your meals or you will end up snacking on junk food just to get though the day.

Take the information and have fun with it. Be willing to step out of your comfort zone and find a new healthier comfort zone.

Chapter 9
Recipes

You will find easy to prepare healthy recipes for everyday cooking. I realize this will never work if it takes hours to prepare meals. Each of the recipes is tried and tested to provide pleasure for your taste buds and health for your body.

Don't be afraid to make changes to fit your family's specific needs and desires. Each of the recipes is made with whole, healthy ingredients. You will find recipes that are made with ground buffalo; you can substitute ground turkey for any of these.

Variety will keep you on the right track so I encourage you to try different recipes each week. We have our favorites, but I am always experimenting with new ideas to keep it interesting.

As you go through the salad and soup sections realize as a family we eat most of them as a main course, and leftovers are great for lunches. It saves time in preparation.

The goal is to eat 5-6 healthy meals a day, the meals don't need to be huge, but they need to be consistent. Give your body regular energy and it will function at its best throughout the entire day. Fresh fruits and vegetables make a great afternoon and mid-morning snack especially for those of us who work long days at the office. Keep things simple and you will be able to use them longer.

Enjoy the recipes, change them to meet your needs, but most importantly use them to create better health for you and your family.

Chapter 10
Appetizers and Munchies

7 Layer Mexican Dip
Bean and Buffalo/Turkey Quesadilla
Black Bean Dip
Buffalo Chicken Tenders
Chicken Vegetable Quesadillas
Creamy Vegetable Dip
Curry Vegetable Dip
Fresh Salsa
Fruit Salsa
Garlic Whole Wheat Pita Chips
Guacamole
Grilled Chicken Quesadillas
Lemon Curry Dip
Salmon Balls
Southwest Vegetable or Corn Chip Dip
Spinach Artichoke Dip
Stuffed Mushrooms
Tomato and Basil Stuffed Mushrooms
Whole Wheat Tortilla Chips

7 Layer Mexican Dip

Prep time: 30 minutes **Chilling Time:** 0-2 hours
Servings: 6

1 can fat free refried beans
1 cup fat free sour cream
1 large avocado
1 tablespoon chili powder
2 teaspoon cumin
½ teaspoon salt
1 teaspoon pepper
½ cup green onions
1 can green chilies
1 can chopped black olives
1 cup tomatoes (chopped)
1½ cup fat free grated cheddar cheese
1½ cup fat free grated mozzarella cheese

Make avocado layer by mashing avocados and adding sour cream, chili powder, cumin, salt, and pepper, mix thoroughly. On a medium size platter spread a layer of refried beans, top with avocado mix, sprinkle green onions, green chilies, black olives and tomatoes. Sprinkle with cheese and serve with corn chips.

Bean and Buffalo/Turkey Quesadilla

Prep Time: 30 minutes   **Cooking Time:** 10-15 minutes
Servings: 4-8

1 pound ground buffalo or turkey
1 small onion
1 tablespoon canola oil
1 teaspoon salt
1 teaspoon pepper
½ teaspoon garlic salt
1 tablespoon chili powder
2 teaspoon cumin
2-3 tablespoon water
1 can fat free refried beans
1 cup fat free grated cheddar cheese
1 c fat free grated mozzarella cheese
8 whole wheat tortilla shells
Guacamole and Salsa (optional)

Sauté onions in canola oil until clear and tender, add meat, crumble and brown. Add spices and water. Cook for 10-15 minutes to blend flavors. Heat large frying pan over medium heat. Place one tortilla in pan, spread ¼ of beans on tortilla, sprinkle with cheddar cheese, and meat. Sprinkle with mozzarella cheese and top with another tortilla shell. Allow to cook until slightly browned on both sides (turning only once). Cook remaining shells as directed above. Cut each quesadilla into 8 pieces and serve with salsa and guacamole.

Black Bean Dip

Prep Time: 10 minutes **Chilling Time:** 2 Hours
Servings: 6

1 can black beans
1 cup salsa
¼ cup cilantro (chopped)
½ cup nonfat sour cream
¼ cup nonfat plain yogurt
1 tablespoon Worcestershire Sauce
8 shakes Tabasco sauce (optional)
Pita or corn chips (optional)
Blend in food processor until smooth, chill for 2 hours to blend flavors. Serve with pita or corn chips if desired.

Buffalo Chicken Tenders

Prep Time: 20 minutes   **Cooking Time:** 25 Minutes
Servings: 4

2 large chicken breasts
¾ cup egg beaters (6 egg whites)
¼ cup fat free milk
1 cup whole wheat flour
1 teaspoon salt
½ teaspoon pepper
cooking oil spray
1/3 cup Franks hot sauce
2 tablespoon melted Benecol (add more if you like it mild

Preheat oven to 400° or Foreman Grill to 375°. Cut chicken in strips. Mix eggbeaters and milk together in shallow bowl. Mix flour, salt and pepper in large plastic bag. Dredge chicken with eggs and coat with flour mix. Spray with cooking spray and place on sprayed baking sheet. If baking in oven, bake for 25 minutes, if grilling place on sprayed grill and cook for 8 minutes. In large bowl mix Franks sauce and Benecol. Toss chicken with sauce. Serve.

Chicken Vegetable Quesadillas

Prep Time: 30 minutes   Cooking Time: 10 Minutes
Servings: 4-8

2 Chicken Breasts
1 cup red onion (chopped)
2 cloves garlic (minced)
2 tablespoon lime juice
1 can corn
1 zucchini sliced
1 cup salsa
½ sweet red pepper (sliced)
1 can green chilies (chopped)
1 teaspoon dried oregano
1½ teaspoon cumin
½ teaspoon salt
½ teaspoon cayenne pepper
8 whole wheat flour tortillas
1 cup fat free grated cheddar cheese
1 cup fat free grated mozzarella cheese
Salsa and guacamole (optional)

Cut chicken into ½ inch cubes. Spray skillet with cooking oil spray. Over medium heat, cook chicken, onion, garlic and lime juice. Add corn, zucchini, salsa, peppers, chilies, and spices. Cover and simmer until vegetables are tender. Warm a frying pan over medium heat. Place one tortilla in pan and sprinkle with ¼ cup cheddar cheese, cover cheese with chicken/vegetable filling and sprinkle with ¼ cup mozzarella cheese, top with another tortilla. Cook until light brown on both sides, turning once. Cook remaining quesadillas. Cut each into 8 pieces and serve with salsa and guacamole if desired.

Creamy Vegetable Dip

Prep Time: 10 minutes   **Chilling Time:** 2 hours
Servings: 6

1 cup fat free sour cream
1 tablespoon apple cider vinegar
2 cloves garlic, (minced)
1½ tablespoon Dijon mustard
1 tablespoon honey
1 tablespoon extra virgin olive oil
½ teaspoon salt
½ teaspoon pepper
½ teaspoon parsley
½ teaspoon tarragon
½ teaspoon chives
½ teaspoon thyme
½ teaspoon Tabasco sauce

Blend together all ingredients and chill for 2 hours prior to serving. Serve with fresh cut up vegetables, broccoli, cauliflower, sweet peppers, carrots, celery, etc.

Curry Vegetable Dip

Prep time: 10 minutes **Chilling Time:** 2-4 hours
Servings: 4-6

2 cup fat free mayonnaise
½ cup fat free sour cream
¼ teaspoon turmeric
1 tablespoon curry powder
½ teaspoon garlic powder
4 teaspoon honey
1 teaspoon salt
2 teaspoon lemon juice
¼ cup minced parsley

Mix ingredients together. Refrigerate for several hours or overnight. For dipping cauliflower, cherry tomatoes, green onions, shrimp, celery, carrot sticks, and green pepper sticks.

Fresh Salsa

Prep time: 30 minutes   **Chilling Time:** 2 hours
Servings: 6

6 ripe tomatoes (diced)
1 white onion (diced)
3-5 Anaheim peppers (diced)
2 cloves garlic (minced)
2 jalapeno peppers (minced)
¼ cup chopped fresh cilantro (optional)
1 tablespoon lime juice
1 teaspoon pepper
1½ teaspoon salt

Combine the ingredients and allow flavors to blend for 2 hour. Store in refrigerator for up to 1 week.

Fruit Salsa

Prep Time: 30 minutes   **Chilling Time:** 2 hours
Servings: 4

1 medium orange
1 cup strawberries (chopped)
1 cup pomegranate
1 can crushed pineapple
¼ cup green onion (chopped)
½ cup red pepper chopped
1 tablespoon lime juice
1 jalapeno pepper (minced)

Combine all the ingredients in a medium bowl, cover and chill for at least 2 hours.

Garlic Whole Wheat Pita Chips

Prep time: 15 minutes   **Baking Time:** 15 minutes
Servings: 6

8 whole wheat pita bread pockets
Cooking oil spray (I use Pam)
Garlic salt or powder

Preheat oven to 350°. Cut each pita into to 4 pieces, separate layers (for 8 chips from each pocket). Spray both sides with cooking oil. Place sprayed pita on a single layer baking sheet, sprinkle with garlic. Bake for 15 minutes. Store in tightly covered container for up to 2 weeks.

Guacamole

Prep Time: 20 minutes **Chilling Time:** 0-4 hours
Servings: 6

2 large avocados
¼ cup onion (minced)
½ cup tomatoes (chopped)
2 tablespoon fat free mayonnaise
2 tablespoon fat free sour cream
1 teaspoon salt
1 teaspoon pepper
1 teaspoon cumin
1½ teaspoon chili powder
2 tablespoon lemon juice

Mash avocados and add remaining ingredients, allow flavors to bend for 1 hour prior to serving. Store in refrigerator for up to 3 days. May be served with baked corn chips.

Grilled Chicken Quesadillas

Prep Time: 30 minutes   **Cooking Time:** 10 minutes
Servings: 4-8

2 chicken breasts
1 tablespoon chili powder
2 teaspoon cumin
1 teaspoon garlic salt
1 teaspoon onion powder
½ teaspoon black pepper
¼ teaspoon cayenne pepper
½ cup chopped green onions
8 whole wheat tortilla shells
1 cup fat free grated cheddar cheese
1 cup fat free grated mozzarella cheese

Combine spices in a small bowl, rub on all sides of the chicken, let sit for 15 minutes. Preheat barbecue grill or Foreman grill (400°). Grill chicken for 7 minutes per side on barbecue grill or for 7 minutes total on Foreman grill. Allow to cool slightly and cut chicken in to strips. Heat large frying pan over medium heat. Place one tortilla in pan, sprinkle with cheddar cheese, green onions and chicken strips. Sprinkle with mozzarella cheese and top with another tortilla shell. Allow to cook until slightly browned on both sides (turning only once). Cook remaining shells as directed above. Cut each quesadilla into 8 pieces and serve with salsa and guacamole.

Lemon Curry Dip

Prep time: 10 minutes   **Chilling Time:** 2-4 hours
Servings: 4-6

16 oz fat free cottage cheese
½ cup plain nonfat yogurt
2 tablespoon lemon juice
1 tablespoon lemon zest
2 teaspoon curry powder
½ teaspoon cardamom
½ teaspoon cayenne pepper

In food processor blend all ingredients, until smooth and creamy chill for 2 hours to blend flavors.

Salmon Balls

Prep Time: 15 Minutes **Chilling Time:** 1 hour
Servings: 4

8 oz. fat free cream cheese, softened
1 tablespoon lemon juice
1 tablespoon horseradish
15 oz. can boneless, skinless salmon, drained
¼ cup fresh chives (chopped)
½ teaspoon salt
Chopped pecans

Mix together salmon with cream cheese, lemon juice, horseradish, salt, and chives. Refrigerate until firm. Form salmon mixture into ball and roll in pecans. Serve with whole wheat crackers.

Southwest Vegetable or Corn Chip Dip

Prep Time: 10 Minutes   Chilling Time: 1 Hour
Servings: 6-10

2 tablespoon fresh cilantro
1½ tablespoon onion, minced
1 tablespoon fresh chives, chopped
1 tablespoon cumin
1½ tablespoon chili powder
¼ teaspoon salt
2 cup fat free mayonnaise

Combine all the ingredient together, mix well. Chill for 1 hour to blend flavors.

Spinach Artichoke Dip

Prep Time: 15 minutes **Chilling Time:** 2-4 hours
Servings: 4-6

2 cloves garlic
4 green onions
1 package frozen spinach, cooked and drained completely
1 bottle pickled artichokes
1 tablespoon lemon juice
1 teaspoon coriander
1 teaspoon salt
½ teaspoon pepper
5-6 shakes Tabasco sauce
1 cup nonfat sour cream
1 cup nonfat plain yogurt

Mince garlic and onion in food processor. Add spinach and artichokes. Add remaining ingredients and blend until smooth. Serve with baked pita chips.

Stuffed Mushrooms

Prep Time: 15 minutes **Baking Time:** 10 minutes
Servings: 4

24 large mushrooms
2 teaspoon olive oil
½ cup walnuts or pecans (chopped)
¼ cup pomegranate juice
¼ cup raisins
¼ cup whole wheat cracker crumbs
1 cup nonfat cottage cheese
½ teaspoon salt
¼ cup chopped green onions

Preheat oven to 400° Remove stems from the mushrooms and chop the stems. You will need 1 cup of the mushrooms. Put the caps stem side down on a baking sheet sprayed with cooking oil spray. In a large pan, heat the oil over medium heat. Stir in the nuts and cook until lightly toasted. Stir in chopped stems, and juice. Cook over high heat until the stems soften. Put sautéed mixture in a bowl and add remaining ingredients. Bake the mushroom tops for 5 minutes, until they begin to soften. Stuff each mushroom with sautéed mixture, mounding it up a little. Set tops back on baking sheet. Bake for 10-14 minutes, until lightly golden, serve immediately.

Tomato and Basil Stuffed Mushrooms

Prep Time: 30 minutes   **Baking Time:** 10 minutes
Servings: 6

24 large mushrooms
15 sun-dried tomatoes (not packed in oil)
2 cup fresh basil
¼ cup olive oil
1 tablespoon water
½ cup fat free cottage cheese
½ cup whole wheat cracker crumbs
4 cloves garlic (minced)
½ teaspoon salt
½ teaspoon pepper

Reconstitute tomatoes by soaking them in very hot water for about 15 minutes. Remove stems from mushrooms and set aside. Preheat oven to 350°. In a food processor blend together tomatoes, basil, oil water, cottage cheese, garlic, mushroom stems, salt and pepper until smooth add cracker crumbs and blend slightly. Mound the mushroom tops with tomato filling, place on baking sheet. Bake until mushrooms begin to soften approximately 10 minutes. Serve immediately.

Whole Wheat Tortilla Chips

Prep time: 15 minutes   **Baking Time:** 10 minutes
Servings: 6

8 whole wheat Tortillas
Cooking oil spray (I use Pam)
1 teaspoon cinnamon (optional)
¼ cup Stevia (optional)
Salt to taste (optional)

Preheat oven to 350°. Cut each Tortilla into to small wedges. Spray both sides tortilla wedges with cooking oil. Place sprayed tortilla on a single layer baking sheet. For sweet chips, sprinkle with cinnamon and Stevia. For savory chips, sprinkle with salt. Bake for 10 minutes. Store in tightly covered container for up to 2 weeks.

Chapter 11
Soups

5 Bean Soup
Black Bean Soup
Buffalo/Turkey Barley Soup
Buffalo Stew
Chicken Stew
Chicken Vegetable and Whole Wheat Noodle Soup
Chili
French Onion Soup
Fresh Basil Vegetable Soup
Hot and Sour Soup
Italian Vegetable Soup
Old Fashion Tomato Soup
Split Pea Soup
Summer Squash Curry Soup
Taco Soup
Tomato Cabbage Soup
Turkey Vegetable Soup
Vegetable Soup

5 Bean Soup

Prep Time: 1 hour   **Cooking Time:** 2 hours
Servings: 6-8

1 cup dried black beans
1 cup dried kidney beans
1 cup dried brown beans
1 cup dried black eyed peas
1 cup dried lima beans
8-10 cup water
1 medium onion (chopped)
1 tablespoon canola oil
2 cloves garlic (minced)
2 cans stewed tomatoes
1 small can green chilies
1 jalapeno pepper (minced, remove seeds and veins)
6 cup hot water

Check and rinse beans, soak in 8-10 cups of water overnight or at least 6 hours. Drain and rinse beans, return to pot. In a small skillet cook onions in canola oil over medium heat until tender. Add to beans, and remaining ingredients. Simmer for 2 hours or until beans are at desired tenderness.

Black Bean Soup

Prep Time: 30 minutes   **Cooking/Soaking Time:** 8 hours   **Servings:** 6

4 cup dried black beans
2 cans fat free beef broth
2 cans fat free chicken broth
1 onion, chopped
2 cloves garlic, mashed
1 tablespoon cumin
3 tablespoon chopped cilantro
Garnish: baked tortilla chips, fat free grated cheese, chopped green onions, guacamole and fat free sour cream

Sort and rinse beans, soak in 8-10 cups of water overnight or at least 6 hours. Drain and rinse beans, return to pot. Combine all ingredients in a large pot, cover and cook 2 hours on low heat until beans are soft. If desired, puree and place back in the pot and thin to desired consistency with extra broth.

Buffalo or Turkey Barley Soup

Prep Time: 45 Minutes **Simmering Time:** 1 hour
Servings: 6-8

2 pounds ground buffalo (can substitute ground turkey)
1 onion (chopped)
1 bell pepper (chopped)
2 cloves garlic (minced)
1 teaspoon salt
1 teaspoon pepper
1 bay leaf
3 carrots (sliced)
3 stalks celery (chopped)
1 can corn
1 can green beans
1 can kidney beans
2 cans chopped tomatoes
1½ cup barley
1 teaspoon thyme
2 teaspoon oregano
2 teaspoon basil
½–1 cup hot water (as needed)

Brown and crumble meat add onion, pepper, garlic, bay leaf, salt and pepper. Cook until onions are clear. Add carrots, celery, corn, beans, and tomatoes. Simmer 45 minutes. Add barley, and spices and extra water as needed, simmer for additional 15 minutes. Serve.

Buffalo Stew

Prep Time: 20 Minutes   **Cooking Time:** 6 Hours
Servings: 4-6

1 pound cubed buffalo
¼ cup whole wheat flour
salt and pepper to taste
1½ tablespoon Worcestershire sauce
1 onion, chopped
3 carrots, sliced
2 stalks celery, sliced
2 cup mushrooms, quartered
2 cloves garlic, minced
1 bay leaf
1 can beef broth
1 can green beans

Place buffalo into a slow cooker. In a small bowl, mix together the flour, salt and pepper; sprinkle over the stew meat, stirring to coat. Stir in the rest of the ingredients except the beans. Cover and cook on low 6 hours, stirring occasionally. Add the beans in the last hour.

Chicken Stew

Prep Time: 30 minutes   **Simmering Time:** 3 Hours
Servings 6-8

3-4 chicken breasts
2-3 quarts water
2 onions, sliced
4 cup fresh tomatoes, chopped
4 cup corn kernels, cut from cob or 2 cans corn
2 cup cut okra or zucchini
2 cup lima beans
3 tablespoon salt
1 teaspoon pepper
1 tablespoon honey

Cut chicken breast in pieces and simmer, covered, in water (3 quarts if thin stew desired, 2 if thick) until meat falls apart, about 2 hours. Remove chicken and set aside to cool. Add onions, okra, tomatoes, lima beans, corn and potatoes to the broth and simmer, uncovered until beans are tender, about 45 minutes. Stir occasionally to prevent scorching. Add chicken, salt, pepper and honey to pot. Heat through. Flavor improves when refrigerated overnight and reheated following day.

Chicken Vegetable and Whole Wheat Noodle Soup

Prep Time: 1 hours   **Simmering Time:** 1 hour
Servings: 6

3 chicken breasts
1 onion (chopped)
1 tablespoon canola oil
3 stalks celery (chopped)
3 carrots (sliced)
1 teaspoon salt
1 teaspoon pepper
1 teaspoon thyme
1 teaspoon rosemary
4 cans fat free chicken broth
1 batch whole wheat noodles (see recipe for whole wheat noodles) or one package whole wheat noodles
Water as needed

Use oil to sauté onions in large pot until tender. Salt and pepper chicken breast and add to onions. Cook until slightly browned and cooked through, approximately 10 minutes per side on medium heat. Add chicken broth to clean bottom of pan. (the brown rouge will give the soup a richer flavor). Add vegetables and spices. Simmer for 45 minutes. Bring to a full boil and add noodles and additional water as needed. Cook for approximately 15 minutes or until noodles are tender. Serve with salad and bread.

Chili

Prep Time: 30 minutes   **Simmering Time:** 1 Hour
Servings 6-8

2 pounds ground turkey
1 onion, chopped
2 to 3 tablespoon garlic, minced
1 cup chopped green pepper
1 cup chopped red pepper
1 cup chopped celery
1 to 2 finely chopped hot peppers
1 teaspoon salt
1 teaspoon pepper
1 tablespoon crumbled dried oregano
2 tablespoon chili powder
2 tablespoon ground cumin
3 cup tomatoes,chopped
1 can fat free beef broth
2 cup kidney beans, drained

Sauté ground meat, chopped onions and garlic until brown. Add remaining ingredients. Simmer for 1 hour.

French Onion Soup

Prep Time: 30 **Simmering Time:** 20 minutes
Servings: 4

2 large onions, sliced
¼ cup Smart Balance or canola oil
3 cans fat free beef broth
1 tablespoon Worcestershire sauce
Dash of pepper
4 slices whole wheat bread, toasted
Grated fat free mozzarella cheese

In large saucepan, cook onions in smart balance until tender. Add beef broth, Worcestershire sauce and pepper. Cover and simmer for 20 to 25 minutes to blend flavors. To serve, top each serving with a slice of toasted bread and sprinkle with cheese. Place under broiler until cheese is bubbly.

Fresh Basil Vegetable Soup

Prep Time: 30 Minutes **Simmering Time:** 30 Minutes
Servings 6-8

3 tablespoon Smart Balance
1 onion, chopped
1 stalk celery, sliced
1 carrot, sliced
2 tomatoes
2 cans chicken or beef broth
3 tablespoon coarsely chopped fresh basil or 1 teaspoon dry basil
½ head cauliflower, broken into flowerets
2 small zucchini, sliced
½ pound fresh green peas, shelled
Salt and pepper

Add Smart Balance to a 5-quart pan over medium heat. Add onion, celery and carrot; cook stirring occasionally until vegetables are soft, but not brown (about 10 minutes. Meanwhile peel and dice tomatoes; you should have 2 cups. Add tomatoes, broth and basil to pan. Bring to a boil, then cover and simmer for 15 minutes. Add cauliflower and zucchini and simmer for 10 more minutes. Add peas and simmer for another 5 minutes or until all vegetables are tender. Season to taste with salt and pepper.

Hot and Sour Soup

Prep Time: 30 Minutes   **Simmering Time:** 13 minutes
Servings: 6

3–4 dried mushrooms
1 cup hot water
2 bean curd cakes
1 scallion (chopped)
2 egg whites
2 tablespoon cornstarch
1/3 cup cold water
Few drops sesame oil
2 cans chicken broth
1 cup mushroom soaking liquid
1 tablespoon sherry
2 tablespoon white vinegar
¾ teaspoon salt (optional)
¼ teaspoon pepper
Tabasco sauce to taste
1 tablespoon soy sauce

Soak dried mushrooms in 1 cup hot water. Reserve soaking liquid. Sliver mushrooms and bean curd. Mince scallion. Beat egg whites lightly. Blend cornstarch and cold water to a paste. Bring stock and mushroom soaking liquid to a boil. Add mushrooms and simmer covered for 10 minutes. Add bean curd and simmer, covered 3 more minutes. Stir in sherry, vinegar, salt, soy sauce and pepper. Thicken with cornstarch paste. Slowly add beaten egg stirring once or twice. Remove from heat. Sprinkle with sesame oil and minced scallion. Add Tabasco sauce to taste.

Italian Vegetable Soup

Prep Time: 30 minutes   **Simmering Time:** 40 minutes
Servings 6-8

1 pound ground buffalo or turkey
2 celery stalks (sliced)
2 cloves garlic (minced)
1 (15 oz.) can tomato sauce
1 tablespoon dried Italian seasoning
1 teaspoon salt
½ teaspoon black pepper
1 medium onion (diced)
1 cup carrots, (sliced)
2 cans stewed tomatoes
1 can tomato sauce
1 can red kidney beans
1 can fat free beef broth
2 cup whole wheat noodles
1 can green beans
2 cup cabbage (shredded)
2-3 tablespoon fresh basil
1 tablespoon fresh oregano

Brown meat and onions in large heavy kettle; drain. Add all the ingredients except cabbage, green beans and noodles and fresh herbs. Bring to a boil. Lower heat; cover and simmer 20 minutes. Add cabbage, green beans and noodles; bring to a boil and simmer until vegetables are tender, add herbs and simmer for 10 minutes. If you prefer a thinner soup, add additional water or broth.

Old Fashion Tomato Soup

Prep Time: 30 minutes **Simmering Time:** 30 minutes
Servings: 6-8

¼ cup Benecol or Smart Balance
2 tablespoon olive oil
1 large onion, (sliced)
2 sprigs fresh thyme or ½ teaspoon dried thyme
4 fresh basil leaves or ½ teaspoon dried basil
1 teaspoon salt
½ teaspoon pepper
2½ pounds diced fresh ripe tomatoes or 2 16 oz cans tomatoes
1 small can tomato paste
¼ cup whole wheat flour
2 cans fat free chicken broth
1 teaspoon honey
1 c fat free milk
8 oz package fat free cream cheese

In a large pan, heat smart balance and olive oil over medium heat. Add onions and seasonings. Cook, stirring occasionally, until the onion is soft. Add the tomatoes and paste. Stir to blend. Simmer 10 minutes. Place the flour in a small mixing bowl and stir in ¼ cup chicken broth. Stir into the tomato mixture. Add the remaining broth. Simmer 30 minutes, stirring frequently. Allow mixture to cool and run through sieve or food processor. Return the pureed mixture to the pot. Add the honey, milk and cream cheese. Heat through, stirring occasionally.

Split Pea Soup

Prep Time: 30 Minutes   **Cooking Time:** 1½ hours
Servings: 4

6 cup water
1½ cup split peas (washed)
½ cup onion (chopped)
3 carrots (sliced)
3 stalks celery, (chopped)
2 teaspoon salt
1 bay leaf

Bring peas to a boil for 3 minutes, reduce heat and simmer until tender, 45 to 50 minutes. Add vegetables and simmer until tender, 25 minutes. Add water as needed. Remove bay leaf. Puree to thicken the soup.

Summer Squash Curry Soup

Prep Time: 15 Minutes   **Cooking Time:** 20 Minutes
Servings: 6

2 pounds yellow squash
2 tablespoon Benecol
1 cup chopped onion
1 teaspoon curry powder
2 Cans chicken broth

Finely chop or coarsely grate yellow summer squash. Sauté onions until golden in benecol. Add curry powder to onions. Sauté onions and curry about one minute more. Add squash to onions and sauté a few minutes. Add chicken broth and cook gently until squash is tender. Puree in blender. Serve either hot or cold.

Taco Soup

Prep Time: 30 Minutes   Simmering Time: 1 Hour
Servings 6-8

2 pounds ground turkey or buffalo
1 onion, chopped
1 pkg. taco seasoning mix
4 (16 oz.) cans tomatoes
1 (16 oz.) can pinto beans
1 (16 oz.) can red kidney beans
1 (4 oz.) can green chilies, chopped
1 teaspoon salt
2 tablespoon Chili powder

Sauté ground meat and chopped onions until brown. Add remaining ingredients. Simmer for 1 hour. Top with grated fat free Cheddar cheese.

Tomato Cabbage Soup

Prep Time: 30 minutes **Simmering Time:** 30 Minutes
Servings: 4-6

1 large can tomato juice
½ head cabbage
5 beef bouillon cubes
1 cup celery, chopped
1 green pepper, Chopped
1 small onion, chopped
2 cup water
Salt and pepper to taste

Combine all ingredients and bring to a boil. Simmer for ½ hour.

Turkey Vegetable Soup

Prep Time: 30 Minutes   **Simmering Time:** 40 Minutes
Servings 6-8

1 pound ground turkey
2 stalks celery (sliced)
2 cloves garlic (minced)
1 can tomato sauce
2 cup water
1 tablespoon dried parsley flakes
1 teaspoon thyme
1 teaspoon salt
2 cup cabbage (shredded)
1 medium onion (diced)
3 carrots (sliced)
1 can tomatoes
1 can kidney beans
1 can corn
1 can green beans
1 teaspoon black pepper

Brown meat in large heavy kettle; drain. Add all the ingredients except cabbage and barley. Bring to a boil. Lower heat; cover and simmer 20 minutes. Add cabbage and barley; bring to a boil and simmer until vegetables are tender.

Vegetable Soup

**Prep Time: 1 hour   Simmering Time: 1½ hour
Servings: 6-8**

3 large cans whole tomatoes
2 large cans chicken broth
1 cup onion (chopped)
1 cup celery (chopped)
2 bay leaves
1 tablespoon basil
2 teaspoon salt
1 teaspoon pepper
4 cup cabbage (coarsely chopped)
2 cup cauliflower cut into small pieces
Parsley
1 can corn
2 cup sliced carrots
2 cup sliced zucchini

Place Tomatoes in a large pot with chicken broth. Bring to a boil. Add remaining vegetables and spices, except 2 teaspoon of basil. Cover and simmer for 1½ hours. Add remaining basil leaves, simmer 5 minutes longer.

Chapter 12
Salads

Avocado Salmon Salad
Blueberry Fruit Salad
Broccoli Pecan Salad
Broccoli Salad
Caesar Salad
Garlic Croutons
Chicken Apple Salad
Chicken Cabbage Salad
Chicken Fajita Salad
Chicken Macadamia Salad
Chinese Coleslaw
Chinese Tuna Salad
Coleslaw
Creamy Coleslaw
Fresh Salmon Salad
Fruit Bowl
Fruit Cocktail
Fruit Kabobs
Fruit Salad
Hot Chicken Lettuce Salad
Lemon Chicken Salad
Mushroom Spinach Salad

Peanut Salad
Salmon Pasta Salad
Southwest Chicken Salad
Southwest Salmon Salad
Spinach Red Onion Salad
Spinach Salad
Strawberry Papaya Salad
Sweet Potato Salad
Tomato Cottage Cheese Salad
Tomato Tuna Salad
Tomato Rice Salad
Tuna Fruit Salad
Vegetable Pasta Salad
Vegetable Salmon Salad
Dijon Salad Dressing
French Dressing
Great Garlic Dressing
Honey Mustard Dressing
Honey Poppy Seed Dressing
Lime Poppy Seed Dressing
Tarragon Twist Salad Dressing

Avocado Salmon Salad
Prep Time: 30 Minutes   Servings: 4-6

3 large avocados
Lettuce
1 (15 oz.) can salmon, chilled
2 tablespoon sliced green onions
2 tablespoon sliced celery
1/3 cup oil
1½ tablespoon lemon juice
1 clove of garlic, minced
1/8 teaspoon dry mustard
¼ teaspoon salt
Dash of pepper
1½ teaspoon minced parsley

Halve, pit and peel avocados. Arrange on lettuce lined plates. Drain salmon; separate into chunks. Toss salmon lightly with green onion and celery. Fill avocados with salmon mixture. Combine remaining ingredients in jar with tight fitting lid; cover. Shake jar vigorously. Drizzle over salmon mixture.

Blueberry Fruit Salad
Prep Time: 15 Minutes   Servings: 4

2 bananas
2 pears, sliced
2 cup strawberries, sliced
2 cans mandarin oranges (drained)
2 cup blueberries

Mix together and refrigerate.

Broccoli Pecan Salad
Prep Time: 30 Minutes   Servings: 4-6

3 cup broccoli
1 cup pecans
1 cup celery
½ cup green onion
1 cup zucchini
Fat free mayonnaise
Salt and pepper to taste

Cut all ingredients in small pieces; salt and pepper to taste, add mayonnaise to taste.

Broccoli Salad

Prep Time: 15 Minutes **Chilling Time:** 1-3 hours
Servings: 6-8

1 head broccoli
½ red onion
10 to 12 slices of cooked turkey bacon
½ to 1 cup raisins
1 cup mayonnaise
½ cup honey
2 tablespoon vinegar

Chop broccoli, onion and bacon in small pieces, mix all together with the raisins. Mix the mayonnaise, honey and viegar to make dressing and put on 1 to 3 hours before serving. Don't put dressing on earlier than 3 hours.

Caesar Salad

Prep Time: 15 minutes   **Servings** 4

2 clove garlic
4 tablespoon olive oil
4 tablespoon fresh lemon juice
1 tablespoon Dijon mustard
2 heads romaine lettuce
Pepper

Place clove garlic in large bowl and crush with fork. Add olive oil and stir briskly. Discard garlic. Add lemon juice and Dijon mustard, and combine with fork; whip. Wash and thoroughly dry lettuce. Break into bite size pieces, discarding heaviest part of the stalk. Add to bowl and toss thoroughly in dressing. Add Garlic Croutons (see below) and pepper to taste. Toss again.

Garlic Croutons

Prep Time: 15 minutes **Cooking Time:** 10 minutes
Servings 4

2 slices whole grain bread
1 tablespoon olive oil
2 teaspoon garlic, minced

Cut bread into small cubes. In small skillet, heat olive oil. Add garlic. Sauté briefly to flavor oil then discard garlic. Add bread pieces and sauté, turning frequently until crisp. Add cubes to salad, soup or vegetable dishes.

Chicken Apple Salad
Prep Time: 15 Minutes   **Servings:** 4

2 cup chicken breast pieces cooked
1 apple, chopped
½ cup celery
2 teaspoon onion
½ cup grapes
½ cup almonds
1 cup fat free mayonnaise
1 teaspoon salt
1 teaspoon curry

Mix all ingredients together and serve, may be refrigerated for 2 hours.

Chicken Cabbage Salad

Prep Time: 15 Minutes **Chilling Time:** Overnight
Servings: 4

½ head cabbage, chopped
4 green onions
4 tablespoon sesame seeds
4 tablespoon sliced almonds
2 chicken breasts, cooked and cut into pieces
¾ cup canola oil
6 tablespoon white vinegar
1 teaspoon pepper
½ teaspoon salt
1 tablespoon honey
Garlic powder

Mix together the above and place in refrigerator to marinate overnight.

Chicken Fajita Salad

Prep Time: 30 Minutes   **Sautéing Time:** 8 minutes
Servings: 4-6

2 tablespoon canola oil, divided
¼ cup lime juice
1 garlic clove, minced
½ teaspoon ground cumin
½ teaspoon oregano
3 chicken breasts, cut into thin strips
1 onion, cut into thin wedges
1 sweet red pepper, cut into thin strips
1 can (7 oz.) chopped green chilies, drained
1 cup whole almonds
Shredded lettuce
3 tomatoes, cut into wedges
1 avocado, sliced

Combine 1 tablespoon oil, lime juice, garlic, cumin and oregano. Toss with chicken; marinate at least 30 minutes. Meanwhile, in a skillet, heat remaining oil on medium-high. Sauté onion 2 minutes. Drain chicken, reserving marinade. Add chicken to skillet; stir-fry until it begins to brown. Add red pepper, chilies and marinade; cook 2 minutes. Stir in almonds. Serve immediately over shredded lettuce and top with tomatoes and avocado.

Chicken Macadamia Salad

Prep Time: 20 Minutes   **Chilling Time:** 30-60 Minutes
Servings: 6-8

3 cup cooked, coarsely chopped chicken breasts (can use canned chicken breasts)
1 can water chestnuts, drained and sliced
¾ cup celery (sliced)
1 cup macadamia nuts (chopped)
2 cup pineapple chunks
2 cup grapes
1 cup fat free mayonnaise
½ teaspoon curry powder
1½ teaspoon soy sauce
1 can mandarin oranges (drained)
lettuce

Place chicken, water chestnuts, celery, and 2/3 cup nuts in large bowl. Mix thoroughly. Add pineapple, grapes, and oranges, mixing lightly. In a separate bowl, mix together mayonnaise, curry powder and soy sauce. Refrigerate until ready to serve. Serve salad on lettuce, garnish with remaining nuts.

Chinese Coleslaw

Prep Time: 20 Minutes   **Chilling Time:** 30-60 Minutes
Servings: 6-8

4 cup cabbage, shredded
½ red onion, thinly sliced
1 stalk celery, chopped
½ cup olive oil
2 tablespoon tarragon Vinegar
1 teaspoon honey
½ teaspoon salt
Tabasco to taste
Paprika

Put the cabbage, onion and celery into a serving bowl. In a small bowl, mix together the olive oil, vinegar, honey, Tabasco, and salt. Pour over the cabbage. Mix well. Sprinkle the top with paprika. Chill for ½–1 hour.

Chinese Tuna Salad

Prep Time: 30 Minutes   **Servings:** 4-6

1 can bean sprouts, drained
2 cans tuna, broken in pieces
1 teaspoon soy sauce
½ cup onion, minced
1 teaspoon salt
1 cup fat free mayonnaise
1 cup celery, minced
½ teaspoon pepper
½ tablespoon chopped parsley
Lettuce

Mix all ingredients together; serve on lettuce.

Coleslaw

**Prep Time: 20 Minutes   Chilling Time: 2-4 Hours
Servings: 4-6**

4 cup cabbage, shredded (you can use any combination of green and red)
1 cup carrot, shredded
½ cup green onions, sliced
3 tablespoon vinegar
3 tablespoon olive oil
2½ tablespoon honey
½ teaspoon dry mustard
½ teaspoon pepper
½ teaspoon salt
5-10 shakes Tabasco sauce

In large bowl combine cabbage, carrots, and onions. Make vinaigrette by combining remaining ingredients in a small bowl. Pour vinaigrette over cabbage and toss to coat. Chill for 2-4 hours.

Creamy Coleslaw

Prep Time: 20 Minutes   **Servings:** 6-8

1 cup fat free mayonnaise
2 tablespoon sugar
2 tablespoon vinegar
1½ teaspoon celery salt
1 head cabbage, shredded
2 large carrots
2 green onions
½ green pepper

Combine mayonnaise with sugar, vinegar and celery salt to make dressing. Shred all other ingredients. Toss together with dressing. Serve immediately.

Fresh Salmon Salad

Prep Time: 20 Minutes **Chilling Time:** 2 Hours
Servings: 4

½ cup fat free mayonnaise
¼ teaspoon dill
1 can salmon, drained and flaked
1 cup chopped celery
¼ cup green onion, chopped
1 cucumber, sliced
1 teaspoon lemon juice
1/8 teaspoon pepper
½ cup toasted walnuts
1 Cantaloupe
Combine all ingredients and chill. Serve with cantaloupe.

Fruit Bowl

Prep Time: 30 Minutes   **Chilling Time:** 30 Minutes
Servings: 12

2 cup chunk pineapple
2 cup water melon balls
2 cup peaches, peeled & sliced
2 cup sliced strawberries
1 cup seedless white grapes
1 fresh pear, peeled & sliced
2 bananas, peeled & sliced
2 oranges, peeled & sliced
Lemon juice
Fruit dressing
¾ cup orange juice
¼ cup canola oil
1 tablespoon honey
½ teaspoon salt

Combine all fruits sprinkling lemon juice over fruit as each is prepared. Chill fruits in tight container. Pour fruit dressing over fruit and toss gently when ready to serve.

Fruit Cocktail

Prep Time: 15 Minutes **Chilling Time:** Overnight
Servings: 8

1 can unsweetened pineapple chunks
1 can unsweetened diced peaches
1 can unsweetened diced pears
1 can unsweetened mandarin oranges
1 pomegranate, seeded
1 banana. sliced
1 apple, diced

Combine all canned ingredients and chill overnight, add fresh fruit and serve. (remember small servings of this, there are still a lot of natural sugars).

Fruit Kabobs

Prep Time: 30 Minutes   Servings: 12

2 oranges
12 seedless grapes
2 thick slices fresh pineapple
1 ripe kiwi fruit
12 strawberries
12 pitted cherries
Watermelon, honeydew, or cantaloupe, cut into 12 (1 inch) cubes

Cut fruit into bite sized slices, cubes, or wedges. Spear fruit on thin skewers. Stand spears in bowl or bucket of crushed ice or use a hollowed out pineapple or watermelon filled with ice, to support the skewers.

Fruit Salad
Prep Time: 20 Minutes   Servings: 4

1 banana, sliced
1 apple, unpeeled, sliced thinly
2 tablespoon lemon juice, sprinkle overfruit
¼ cup orange juice
2 tablespoon fat free mayonnaise
2 tablespoon honey
Shredded salad greens
2 tablespoon chopped peanuts

Blend orange juice, mayonnaise and honey together and pour over fruit. Combine all ingredients and top with peanuts.

Hot Chicken Lettuce Salad

Prep Time: 30 Minutes **Chilling Time:** 15 Minutes
Servings: 4

1 head lettuce
2 chicken breast, cooked and shredded
¼ cup chopped parsley
¼ cup toasted sesame seeds
1/3 cup chopped scallions
¼ cup slivered almonds
Dressing
4 tablespoon vinegar
4 tablespoon honey
1½ teaspoon salt
½ teaspoon ground pepper
¼ cup olive oil

Toss salad ingredients and chill. Add dressing just before serving. Dressing: Heat vinegar, honey, salt and pepper until honey melts. Cool, add oil and whip. Toss with salad.

Lemon Chicken Salad

Prep Time: 15 Minutes   **Chilling Time:** 2 Hours
Servings: 4

½ cup fat free mayonnaise
¼ cup fat free sour cream
1 tablespoon honey
½ teaspoon grated lemon rind
1 tablespoon lemon juice
1 teaspoon ground ginger
¼ teaspoon salt
2 cup cooked, cubed chicken
1 cup sliced seedless green grapes
1 cup sliced celery
½ cup Sliced almonds

Stir together first 7 ingredients. Add chicken, grapes and celery; toss to coat well. Cover, chill at least 2 hours. Serve with sliced almonds.

Mushroom Spinach Salad

Prep Time: 15 Minutes   Servings: 4

1 pound spinach
4 or 5 fresh mushrooms
3 tablespoon fresh Parmesan cheese
Virgin olive oil
Garlic red wine vinegar

Wash and drain spinach. Chop very fine. Slice mushrooms very thin; add to spinach. Add slivered Parmesan cheese. Add olive oil, one teaspoon at a time, tossing until spinach looks wet. Add vinegar to taste. Serve at once.

Peanut Salad

Prep Time: 30 Minutes   **Chilling time:** 15 minutes
Servings: 4-6

¼ cup white wine vinegar
¼ cup salad oil
2 tablespoon honey
Pinch of salt
1½ teaspoon curry powder
1 teaspoon dry mustard
1 head leaf lettuce, torn in bite-size pieces
1½ cup apples, chopped
½ cup peanuts
2 tablespoon sliced green onions

To make dressing combine vinegar, oil, honey, salt, curry powder and mustard in jar. Shake and chill for 15 minutes. Place torn lettuce in large salad bowl; top with apple, peanuts and green onions. Add dressing and toss.

Salmon Pasta Salad

Prep Time: 15 Minutes   **Chilling Time:** 3 Hours
Servings: 4

1 cup hot, cooked whole wheat twist pasta
½ cup red salmon (fresh, cooked, or canned), broken into pieces
¼ cup thinly sliced zucchini
¼ cup thinly sliced celery
¼ cup pimento strips
¼ cup olive oil
1 tablespoon white wine vinegar
½ teaspoon Dijon mustard
½ teaspoon lemon juice
1/8 teaspoon garlic salt
1 egg white
Lettuce leaves

In bowl, combine pasta, salmon, zucchini, celery, and pimento, set aside. In blender container, combine olive oil, vinegar, mustard, lemon juice, salt and egg white, blend until smooth. Pour over salad ingredients. Cover and chill several hours Serve on lettuce leaves.

Southwest Chicken Salad

Prep Time: 30 Minutes   **Chilling Time:** 60 Minutes
Servings: 4-6

2 c shredded cooked chicken (may use canned chicken)
1 head shredded Romaine lettuce
2 tomatoes, chopped
½ red onion, thinly sliced
½ cup fat free mozzarella cheese, shredded
4 oz. can diced green chilies
½ cup shredded jicama
¼ cup chopped cilantro
1 avocado
Dressing
½ cup fat free mayonnaise
2/3 cup fat free sour cream
1 tablespoon ground cumin
Baked blue corn chips

Gently toss the chicken, lettuce, tomatoes, onion, cheese, chilies, jicima, and cilatro and refrigerate for 1 hour or more. Just before serving, cut avocado and add to salad. Combine dressing ingredients and pour over all and garnish with baked blue corn tortilla chips.

Southwest Salmon Salad

Prep Time: 60 Minutes **Cooking Time:** 30 Minutes
Serving: 6

Dressing:
1 garlic clove, minced
1 jalapeno pepper, stemmed
½ cup fresh lime juice
½ cup fresh orange juice
½ D olive oil
2 teaspoon Cajun mustard
1 teaspoon salt
¾ teaspoon ground cumin
1 teaspoon honey

Salsa:
4 green onions, cut into 1/4 in. pieces
2 fresh tomatillos, husks removed, minced
1 plum tomato, halved, cut into 1/4 in. pieces
Salad:
2 bunches watercress, stems trimmed
1 head Romaine lettuce
½ cup fresh cilantro, stems trimmed

4 salmon fillets, halved
½ red bell pepper, pressed flat
½ green bell pepper, pressed flat
Salt and freshly ground pepper
1 jicama, peeled, cut into 2 in. julienne
2 ripe avocados, peeled, seeded, cut into 8 wedges each

For Dressing: Mince garlic and jalapeno in blender or processor. Add lime and orange juices, olive oil, and mustard and blend until smooth. Mix in salt, cumin, and honey.

For Salsa: Combine green onions, tomatillos, and tomato in medium bowl. Mix in ¼ cup dressing.

For Salad: Tear watercress and Romaine into bite-size pieces. Combine with cilantro in large bowl. (Salsa and salad can be prepared 4 hours ahead.)

Place salmon in plastic bag with ¼ cup dressing. Marinate 20 minutes. Prepare grill (medium-high heat) or preheat broiler. Char skin side of peppers until blackened, about 8 minutes. Wrap in paper bag and let stand 10 minutes to steam. Peel and cut 1/4 inch pieces. Add to salsa. Drain salmon and discard marinade. Season with salt and pepper. Grill until cooked through, 2 minutes per side.

Add jicama and remaining dressing to greens and toss to coat. Adjust seasoning. Divide among 4 chilled plates. Garnish each plate with 4 avocado wedges. Remove skin from salmon. Place 2 salmon pieces atop greens on each plate. Spoon salsa over salmon and avocado. Serve immediately.

Spinach Red Onion Salad
Prep Time: 10 minutes   Servings: 4-6

1-2 pounds spinach
1 red onion, very thinly sliced
1 (16 oz.) can mandarin oranges, drained
½ cup slivered almonds
Red Onion Dressing:
¼ cup red onion
½ cup honey
1 teaspoon dry mustard
1 teaspoon salt
1 teaspoon celery seed
1/3 cup vinegar
1 cup canola oil

Combine spinach, onion, mandarin oranges, and almonds to make salad. Combine dressing ingredients and toss with salad.

Spinach Salad

Prep Time: 15 Minutes   Servings 4

1 large bunch spinach or ½ head lettuce, shredded
1 tablespoon minced parsley
4 green onions, chopped
1 cup fresh strawberries (sliced)
¼ cup chopped pecans
Dressing
½ teaspoon salt
2 tablespoon vinegar
¼ cup olive oil
2 tablespoon honey
Dash of pepper

Combine spinach or lettuce, parsley, green onions, strawberries, and pecans to make salad. Combine dressing ingredients. Toss with salad.

Strawberry Papaya Salad

Prep Time: 15 Minutes   **Servings:** 2-4

1/3 cup raspberries
2 teaspoon fresh lime juice
1 tablespoon honey or to taste
2 cup strawberries, hulled and halved
1 papaya, peeled and sliced

In blender or food processor, puree raspberries with lime juice and honey. In serving bowl, mix strawberries and papaya together. Pour puree dressing over fruit, toss gently, and serve immediately.

Sweet Potato Salad

Prep Time: 45 Minutes   **Chilling Time:** 1 Hour
Servings: 6-8

¾ cup fat free mayonnaise
¾ cup nonfat plain yogurt
1½ tablespoon curry powder
½ teaspoon salt
2½ pounds sweet potatoes cooked, peeled, cooled, & cut into chunks
2 Granny Smith apples, cut in ½ inch pieces
1 can juice packed pineapple tidbits, drained
½ cup raisins

Whisk mayo, yogurt, curry and salt in large bowl. Add potatoes, apples, pineapple and raisins. Toss gently to mix and coat. Cover and chill at least 1 hour for flavors to develop, or up to 3 days.

Tomato Cottage Cheese Salad

Prep Time: 20 Minutes   Marinade Time: 5 Hours
Servings: 6

2/3 cup olive oil
¼ cup tarragon vinegar
¼ cup chopped parsley
¼ cup sliced green onions
½ teaspoon thyme or marjoram
1 teaspoon salt
¼ teaspoon pepper
1 clove garlic, minced
6 sm. tomatoes, blanched, peeled
Lettuce
Cottage Cheese

Combined olive oil, vinegar, parsley, green onions, marjoram, salt, pepper and garlic. Dry tomatoes well and place and place in combined mixture. Marinade for at least five hours. Cut an "X" in the top of each tomato so it opens slightly, spoon in cottage cheese and serve on lettuce bed, dribble with extra marinade.

Tomato Tuna Salad
Prep Time: 20 Minutes   Servings: 4

½ cup red onion, diced small
1/3 cup fat free mayonnaise
¼ teaspoon salt
2 cans white tuna (packed in water), drained
½ cup celery, chopped
¼ cup fresh tarragon, chopped
Lettuce
4 ripe tomatoes

Whisk mayonnaise, salt and pepper in medium bowl add tuna, celery, tarragon and onion, stir to combine. Serve on lettuce with tomatoes.

Tomato Rice Salad

Prep Time: 20 Minutes   **Marinade Time:** 30 Minutes
Servings: 6

3 cucumbers, sliced
2 tomatoes, diced
1 bell pepper, chopped
1 bunch green onions, sliced
½ cup soy sauce
6 cup cooked brown rice

Combine cucumbers, tomatoes, green bell pepper and green onions. Add soy sauce and let set for 20-30 minutes, stirring frequently. Serve over cooked rice.

Tuna Fruit Salad

Prep Time: 20 Minutes **Chilling Time:** 2 Hours
Servings: 6

¾ cup fat free mayonnaise
2 tablespoon lemon zest
juice of ½ lemon
2 cans each tuna, drained, chunked
1 cup grapes, cut in half, seeded
4 oranges, peeled, cut in bite-size pieces
1 red apple, unpeeled, cut in bite-size pieces
½ cup chopped walnuts
Salad greens and lemon wedges

Combine mayonnaise, lemon zest and juice. Stir in tuna, grapes, oranges, apples and walnuts. Chill. Serve on salad greens; top with lemon wedges.

Vegetable Pasta Salad

Prep Time: 30 Minutes **Chilling Time:** 4 Hours
Servings 12-16

1½ cup whole wheat pasta
2 cup broccoli flowerets
1 cup cauliflower flowerets
1 cup sliced mushrooms
1 (6 oz.) can artichoke hearts, drained, rinsed & chopped
1 cup sliced ripe olives
½ cup chopped green onion
¼ cup olive oil
¼ cup balsamic vinegar
2 tablespoon fresh basil
2 tablespoon fresh oregano
½ teaspoon salt
½ teaspoon pepper
1 clove garlic, minced
1 avocado, seeded, peeled & sliced
1 tomato, chopped

Cook pasta according to package directions; drain. Rinse with cold water; drain well. In a large bowl combine pasta, broccoli, cauliflower, mushrooms, artichoke hearts, olives and green onion. Toss with olive oil, vinegar and spices. Cover and chill several hours. At serving time, toss vegetable mixture with avocado and tomato.

Vegetable Salmon Salad

Prep Time: 45 Minutes   **Chilling Time:** 1 Hour
Servings: 4-6

1½ pounds thick sliced salmon steaks, cut into bite sized pieces & poached
1 onion
2 cup Chinese pea pods
1 cup red pepper strips, wash & cook until tender
½ cup olive oil
¼ cup white wine vinegar
1 tablespoon lemon juice
1 teaspoon dry mustard
¼ teaspoon crushed basil
Salt and Pepper to taste
Lettuce

To make dressing combine olive oil, vinegar, lemon juice, mustard, basil, salt and pepper and mix well.

Marinate hot salmon and onions in dressing for at least 1 hour. Remove salmon from dressing. Toss pea pods and pepper strips in dressing. Gently toss together salmon, onions, pea pods, and peppers. Serve with reserved dressing on a bed of lettuce.

Dijon Salad Dressing
Prep Time: 10 Minutes

4 tablespoon Dijon mustard
3 tablespoon red wine vinegar
1 tablespoon white vinegar
¼ teaspoon salt
1 to 2 cloves garlic
½ teaspoon basil
¼ teaspoon black pepper
¼ teaspoon hot sauce
1 tablespoon grated onion
½ cup canola oil

Combine mustard and vinegar in blender. Add salt, garlic, basil, black pepper, hot sauce and onion; whirl in blender. With machine running, add oil, 1 tablespoon at a time. Chill. Keeps for several weeks refrigerated.

French Dressing
Prep Time: 10 Minutes   Standing Time: 1 Hour

½ teaspoon paprika
½ teaspoon celery salt
1 teaspoon salt
2 tablespoon honey, melted
½ cup olive oil
¼ cup apple cider vinegar
1 teaspoon chopped parsley
1 onion, minced
1 clove garlic

Add 2 tablespoon of the oil to paprika, celery salt, salt and honey; whisk for 5 minutes. Add 1 tablespoon vinegar and continue to beat. Repeat, alternating oil and vinegar. Add parsley, onion and garlic; let stand 1 hour. Remove garlic and store in refrigerator.

Great Garlic Dressing

Prep Time: 10 Minutes   **Standing Time:** Overnight

2 cloves garlic, minced
½ teaspoon salt
2 tablespoon Dijon mustard
1 teaspoon honey, melted
2 tablespoon vinegar
½ cup olive oil

Mix together and let stand at room temperature overnight.

Honey Mustard Dressing
Prep Time: 10 Minutes

¾ cup fat free mayonnaise
½ tablespoon Dijon mustard
1½ tablespoon honey
½ tablespoon lemon juice
½ tablespoon red wine vinegar
1 teaspoon skim milk

Blend and serve.

Honey Poppy Seed Dressing
Prep Time: 10 Minutes

1 cup honey
1 teaspoon mustard
1 teaspoon paprika
¼ teaspoon salt
2 teaspoon poppy seeds
3 tablespoon vinegar
1 teaspoon lemon juice
1 cup olive oil

Blend everything except oil; add oil, slowly while blending. Blend until smooth.

Lime Poppy Seed Dressing
Prep Time: 10 Minutes

1/3 cup honey
¼ cup olive oil
½ teaspoon lime zest
1½ teaspoon poppy seeds
¼ teaspoon salt

Whisk ingredients together and serve.

Tarragon Twist Salad Dressing

Prep Time: 10 Minutes   Standing Time: Several Hours

¼ cup olive oil
¼ cup water
¼ wine vinegar
1 clove garlic, minced
1 teaspoon tarragon, crumbled
½ teaspoon salt

Combine all ingredients in jar. Shake well to blend. Let stand several hours to blend flavors.

Chapter 13
Breads

Amazing Whole Wheat Bread
Cinnamon Raisin Nut Bread
Citrus Pomegranate Bread
Savory Garlic Bread
Apple Raisin Nut Bread
Banana Nut Bread
Cinnamon Rolls
Orange Rolls
Corn Bread
Ginger Bread
Hamburger Buns
Jalapeno Cornbread
Molasses Rolls
Pumpkin Bread
Zucchini Bread
Apple Oatmeal Muffins
Applesauce Muffins
Blueberry Muffins
Bran Muffins
Carrot Muffins
Cranberry Muffins
Favorite Fruit Muffins
Wheat Germ Muffins
French Toast
Granola
Pancakes
Waffles

Amazing Whole Wheat Bread
Prep Time: 1 ½ hours   **Baking Time:** 35 minutes
Servings: 3 large loafs

10 cup whole wheat flour
3 tablespoon dry yeast (rounded)
2 tablespoon vital wheat gluten (rounded)
1 cup nonfat plain yogurt
5 cup hot water
1 ½ tablespoon salt
½ cup canola oil
½ cup honey
¼ cup molasses
2 cup popcorn flour
2 cup oat flour
2 cup whole wheat flour (more or less)

Stir together 10 C. whole wheat flour, yeast and gluten, add yogurt and water, blend well. Cover with a towel and allow to sponge (mixture will begin rising and look like a sponge. for 10 minutes. Add remaining ingredients except 2 cups whole wheat flour mix well, add remaining flour slowly and just enough to have dough form a ball and clean sides of bowl. Turn out on bread board and knead for 5-10 minutes. Form 3 large loaves put in loaf pans and let rise until doubled. Be sure to let it rise in the pans because it will rise very little in the oven. Bake in 350° oven for 35-40 minutes. Remove from pans and cool on racks. Eat within a week or store in plastic bags in freezer for 60 days. Note: using frozen whole wheat flour makes a nicer texture.

Variations:

Cinnamon Raisin Nut Bread
1 tablespoon cinnamon
1 cup raisins
1 cup finely chopped nuts
½ cup honey
¼ cup Benecol Spread

Combine ingredients and set aside. Roll 1/3 of dough to ½–1 inch thick, spread with filling. Roll up and place in loaf pan. Bake for 35 minutes at 350°.

Citrus Pomegranate Bread
1 cup frozen pomegranate seeds
1 tablespoon orange zest
1 tablespoon lemon zest
2 tablespoon fresh squeezed orange juice
2 tablespoon fresh squeezed lemon juice
½ cup honey

Combine ingredients and set aside. Roll 1/3 of dough to ½–1 inch thick, spread with filling. Roll up and place in loaf pan. Bake for 35 minutes at 350°.

Savory Garlic Bread
1 tablespoon fresh minced garlic
2 teaspoon thyme
1 tablespoon basil
1 tablespoon oregano
2 teaspoon parsley
¼ cup Benecol spread

Combine ingredients and set aside. Roll 1/3 of dough to ½–1 inch thick, spread with filling. Roll up and place in loaf pan. Bake for 35 minutes at 350°.

Apple Raisin Nut Bread

Prep Time: 30 Minutes **Baking Time:** 1 hour
Servings: 12-15

2 egg whites
½ cup Canola oil
1½ cup whole wheat flour
¾ cup honey
1½ teaspoon ground cinnamon
1 teaspoon baking soda
1 teaspoon vanilla
½ teaspoon salt
2 teaspoon baking powder
1 cup chopped walnuts
1 cup raisins
1 cup shredded apples (2 med.)

Combine egg whites, oil, flour, honey, cinnamon, baking soda, vanilla, salt and baking powder in large mixing bowl. Stir until well blended. Stir in nuts, raisins, and apples until stiff batter is formed. Pour into loaf pan sprayed with cooking oil. Bake at 375° for 1 hour.

Banana Nut Bread

Prep Time: 15 Minutes **Baking Time:** 50 Minutes
Servings: 12-15

1½ cup whole wheat flour
2 teaspoon baking powder
¼ teaspoon baking soda
½ teaspoon salt
1 teaspoon cinnamon
1 egg white
1 cup mashed banana (3 medium)
¾ cup honey
¼ cup canola oil
2 teaspoon lemon zest
½ cup chopped pecans

Spray the bottom and ½ inch up to sides of a loaf pan with cooking spray, I use Pam. In mixing bowl combine flour, baking powder, baking soda, cinnamon, and salt. Make a well in the center and set aside. In another bowl combine egg whites, bananas, honey, oil and lemon zest add egg mixture to dry ingredients. Stir just until moist. Fold in nuts. Spoon batter into loaf pan. Bake at 350° for 50-55 minutes. Cool in pan for 10 minutes. Remove from pan and cool on rack.

Cinnamon Rolls

Prep Time: 30 Minutes   **Baking Time:** 20 Minutes
Servings: 24

3 cup whole wheat flour
1½ cup sorghum flour
2 tablespoon yeast
1 cup skim milk
1/3 cup honey
1/3 cup coconut oil
1 teaspoon salt
2 egg whites
3 tablespoon Benecol
1/3 cup honey
2 teaspoon cinnamon

Prepare baking pan by spraying bottom and sides of pan cooking spray like Pam. In mixing bowl combine 2 cup flour and yeast. Set aside. In medium saucepan heat milk, 1/3 cup honey, oil, and salt until very warm. Add milk mixture and egg whites to flour and yeast, mix well. Let sponge for 10 minutes. Add remaining flour and knead for 3-5 minutes. Mix benecol, honey, and cinnamon. Divide dough in ½, roll each ½ in to a rectangle. Spread the honey mixture on dough and roll up, like a jelly roll. Using thread, slice each roll in to 12 equal pieces, place in prepared pan. Cover and let rise until double. Bake at 375° for 20-25 minutes or until golden.

Orange Rolls (variation of cinnamon rolls)
Prep Time: 30 Minutes   **Baking Time:** 20 Minutes
Servings: 24

3 tablespoon benecol
¼ cup honey
¼ cup fresh squeezed orange juice
2 teaspoon orange zest

Mix and spread on cinnamon roll dough in place of cinnamon filling. Follow that recipe otherwise.

Corn Bread

Prep Time: 15 Minutes **Baking Time:** 20-25 Minutes
Servings: 6-8

1 ¼ cup whole wheat flour
½ cup popcorn flour
¾ cup stone ground cornmeal
¼ cup honey
2 teaspoon baking powder
½ teaspoon salt
1 cup skim milk
¼ cup canola oil
2 egg whites

Heat oven to 400°. Spray an 8 inch pan with cooking spray (Pam). Combine dry ingredients. Stir in milk, oil, honey and egg whites, mixing just until dry ingredients are moistened. Pour batter into pan. Bake for 20-25 minutes or until light golden brown and wooden pick inserted in center comes out clean. Serve warm.

Ginger Bread

Prep Time: 20 Minutes   **Baking Time:** 30-40 Minutes
Servings: 12-15

1 egg white
1 cup molasses
2½ cup whole wheat flour
½ cup honey
½ cup canola oil
1 teaspoon ginger
1 teaspoon cinnamon
1/8 teaspoon cloves
1½ teaspoon baking soda
1 cup hot water

Beat egg whites until fluffy, add molasses. Blend in flour 1 cup at a time. Add oil and honey, followed by spices and baking soda. Add 1 cup hot water last and mix well on low speed. Pour into 9x13 pan sprayed with cooking spray and bake 30-40 minutes at 350° Cool slightly and serve lukewarm.

Hamburger Buns

Prep Time: 30 Minutes   **Baking Time:** 15-20 Minutes
Servings: 6-8

½ cup skim milk
½ cup water
¼ cup honey
1 teaspoon salt
4 tablespoon coconut oil
1 egg white
3 tablespoon yeast, softened in ¼ cup warm water
2½ cup whole wheat flour
1 cup popcorn flour

Scald liquid, add honey, salt and oil. Cool. Add egg white and yeast. Stir in flour. Shape into buns. Let rise double and bake at 425° for 15-20 minutes.

Jalapeno Cornbread

Prep Time: 10 Minutes **Baking Time:** 35 Minutes
Servings: 6-8

1 cup cornmeal
1 cup whole wheat flour
1 tablespoon baking powder
¾ teaspoon salt
½ cup egg beaters
1 cup skim milk
2 tablespoon canola oil
1 cup whole kernel corn
1 jalapeno pepper, chopped
3 tablespoon chopped pimiento

Combine all ingredients; mixing well. Pour batter into a greased 8 inch square pan. Bake at 350° for 35 minutes or until lightly browned.

Molasses Rolls

Prep Time: 40 Minutes   **Baking Time:** 12 Minutes
Servings: 25

3 cup whole wheat flour
1 cup popcorn flour
2 tablespoon yeast
1 cup skim milk
1/3 cup molasses
¼ cup coconut oil
1 teaspoon salt
2 egg whites
¾ cup rolled oats

Prepare baking pans by spraying bottom and sides. In mixing bowl stir together 2 cup whole wheat flour, and yeast. In medium sauce pan heat and stir the milk, molasses, oil, and salt, until very warm. Add milk mixture to flour and yeast, mix well. Let sponge for 10 minutes. Add egg whites and remaining flours and oats, with enough flour to make a stiff dough. Knead for 6-8 minutes. Allow dough to rest for 5 minutes, shape rolls into small balls and place in baking pan. Allow to rise to double and bake at 375° for 12-15 minutes. Remove from pan and cool on racks.

Pumpkin Bread

Prep Time: 20 Minutes   **Baking Time:** 50-60 Minutes
Servings: 12-15

1½ cup whole wheat flour
1 cup honey
2 teaspoon baking soda
1 cup pumpkin puree
½ cup canola oil
2 egg whites
¼ cup water
¼ teaspoon nutmeg
¼ teaspoon cinnamon
¼ teaspoon allspice
½ cup chopped nuts
½ cup raisins

Preheat oven to 350°. Sift together the flour and baking soda. Mix the pumpkin, oil, honey, egg whites, water, and spices together. Then combine with the flour mixture. Do not mix too thoroughly, mixture should be slightly lumpy. Stir in the nuts and raisins. Pour into a loaf pan sprayed with Pam. Bake 50-60 minutes at 350°.

Zucchini Bread

Prep Time: 30 Minutes **Baking Time:** 1 Hour
Servings: 12-15

1 egg white
1/3 cup canola oil
¾ cup honey
¾ cup grated zucchini
1 teaspoon vanilla
½ cup chopped nuts (optional)
1 cup whole wheat flour
½ teaspoon baking soda
½ teaspoon salt
1 teaspoon cinnamon
½ teaspoon baking powder

Preheat oven at 325°. Beat egg whites until light. Add oil, honey, zucchini and nuts, if desired. Combine flour, baking soda, salt, cinnamon, and baking powder. Add egg mixture and mix until well blended. Pour batter in loaf pan. Bake at 325° for 1 hour.

Apple Oatmeal Muffins

Prep Time: 25 Minutes **Baking Time:** 20-25 Minutes
Servings: 8-10

1¼ cup whole wheat flour
1 cup quick-cooking rolled oats
2 teaspoon baking powder
1 teaspoon baking soda
1½ teaspoon cinnamon
2 egg whites
1 cup frozen, unsweetened apple juice concentrate, thawed
2 c. chopped apples

Combine flour, oats, baking powder, baking soda, and cinnamon. In separate bowl, combine egg white, apple juice concentrate and chopped apples. Add liquid mixture to dry ingredients, blend until just moistened. Divide batter into muffin tins that have been sprayed with nonstick vegetable coating. Bake at 350° for 20 to 25 minutes.

Applesauce Muffins

Prep Time: 15 Minutes **Baking Time:** 20-25 Minutes
Servings: 8

1 egg white
2 tablespoon canola oil
1½ cup unsweetened applesauce
1½ cup whole wheat pastry flour
½ cup bran (wheat or oat, or mixed)
¾ teaspoon baking soda
2 teaspoon baking powder
1 teaspoon cinnamon
1 teaspoon nutmeg
¾ cup raisins
1 tablespoon honey

Beat together eggbeaters, oil, and applesauce. Add flours and bran, baking soda, baking powder, and spices; beat well. Stir in raisins. Spoon batter into sprayed and floured muffin wells or Teflon muffin pan. Bake at 375° for 20-25 minutes or until firm to the touch and browned. Remove from pan and cool on wire racks.

Blueberry Muffins

Prep Time: 20 Minutes   **Baking Time:** 25 Minutes
Servings 12

1¼ cup bran cereal
1¼ cup skim milk
1½ cup whole wheat pastry flour
½ cup wheat germ
½ cup chopped pecans
1 tablespoon baking powder
Pinch of salt
1 egg white
¼ cup olive oil
¼ cup maple syrup or honey
¼ cup molasses
1 pint fresh blueberries

Measure the bran into a bowl with the milk. Let stand until the bran is softened. In a large mixing bowl, combine the flour, wheat germ, pecans, baking powder, and salt. In a medium mixing bowl, beat the egg whites, oil, maple syrup and molasses together until well mixed. Combine the bran and egg white mixture quickly with the flour, using several swift strokes. Gently fold in the blueberries and divide the batter evenly among 12 well-greased 1½ inch muffin tins. Bake in a preheated 400° oven for 25 minutes.

Bran Muffins

Prep Time: 30 Minutes **Baking Time:** 15-20 Minutes
Servings: 8

½ cup unprocessed bran
½ cup boiling water
1 egg white
½ cup Molasses
¼ cup canola oil
1½ teaspoon vanilla extract
1 c. nonfat yogurt
1¼ teaspoon baking soda
¾ cup raisins
1/3 cup chopped pecans
1¼ cup whole wheat flour
¼ teaspoon salt

Combine bran and boiling water in a small bowl, set aside. Combine egg white, molasses, oil and vanilla in a medium mixing bowl. Combine yogurt and soda, stir in well; add yogurt mixture, raisins and chopped pecans to molasses mixture, mixing well. Combine whole wheat flour, bran and salt in a large mixing bowl. Add yogurt mixture and bran and water mixture, stirring just until moistened. Spoon into sprayed muffin pan. Bake at 350° degrees for 15 or 20 minutes.

Carrot Muffins

Prep Time: 15 Minutes **Baking Time:** 20-25 Minutes
Servings: 12

2 cup whole wheat flour
¼ cup honey
1 tablespoon baking powder
1 teaspoon salt
1 cup grated raw carrots
¾ cup skim milk
½ cup chopped nuts
¼ cup canola oil
1 egg white
2 teaspoon grated orange peel

Sift together flour, baking powder and salt. Mix together carrot, milk, honey, nuts, oil, egg white and orange peel. Add carrot mixture all at once to flour mixture, stirring just until dry ingredients are moistened. Fill greased muffin cups 2/3 full. Bake at 425° for 20-25 minutes.

Cranberry Muffins

Prep Time: 20 Minutes **Baking Time:** 30 minutes
Servings: 12

3 cup whole wheat flour
3 teaspoon baking powder
1 teaspoon baking soda
½ teaspoon salt
2 cup fat free sour cream
2/3 cup skim milk
½ cup honey
¼ cup canola oil
½ teaspoon almond extract
2 egg whites
1½ cup fresh or frozen cranberries, chopped
2 tablespoon sliced blanched almonds

Prepare muffin tins by spraying with cooking oil and lightly flouring with whole wheat flour. Preheat oven to 375° In large bowl with a fork, mix dry ingredients. In medium bowl, beat sour cream, milk, honey, oil, almond extract and egg whites until blended. Stir into the flour mixture just until flour is moistened. With rubber spatula, gently fold in cranberries. Spoon batter into muffin pan; sprinkle with sliced almonds. Bake 30 minutes or until toothpick inserted in center comes out clean. Serve warm or cool on rack to serve later.

Favorite Fruit Muffins

Prep Time: 30 Minutes **Baking Time:** 35 Minutes
Servings: 8

2¼ cup whole wheat flour
¾ cup honey
1 tablespoon cinnamon
2 teaspoon baking soda
½ teaspoon salt
2 cup grated carrot
1 apple, shredded
½ cup unsweetened coconut
½ cup raisins
½ cup pecans or walnuts
1 (8 oz.) can unsweetened crushed pineapple, drained
3 egg whites
1 cup Canola oil
1 teaspoon pure vanilla extract

Heat oven to 350°. Spray muffin cups or use paper liners. Sift the flour, cinnamon, baking soda and salt into a large bowl. Stir in the carrots, apple, coconut, raisins, nuts and pineapple. In a separate bowl whisk the egg whites together with the oil, honey, and vanilla. Pour the mixture into the bowl with the dry ingredients; blend well. Spoon batter into muffin cups, filling almost to the top. Bake until a wooden pick inserted in the center comes out clean about 35 minutes. Cool muffins in the pan for 10 minutes, then turn out onto a wire rack to finish cooling. They are best when allowed to ripen for 24 hours before serving.

Wheat Germ Muffins

Prep Time: 10 Minutes   **Baking Time:** 15-20 Minutes
Servings: 12

1 cup whole wheat flour
1 teaspoon salt
3 teaspoon baking powder
¼ cup nonfat powdered milk
1 cup wheat germ
1 cup Skim milk
2 egg whites
¼ cup honey or molasses
2 tablespoon canola oil
½ cup raisins (optional)

Combine in mixing bowl the flour, salt, baking powder, and powdered milk. Add and stir only until moist the wheat germ, milk, egg whites, honey or molasses, and oil. Fill paper baking cups or well greased muffin pans two thirds full. Bake at 400° for 15 to 20 minutes, or until brown. ½ cup raisins may be added with the wheat germ.

French Toast

Prep Time: 3 Minutes   **Cooking Time:** 5 Minutes
Servings: 5

½ cup Eggbeaters
¼ cup skim milk
¼ teaspoon vanilla
¼ teaspoon cinnamon
5 slices whole wheat bread

Prepare skillet, but heating for 2-3 minutes. In shallow bowl, beat together eggs, milk, vanilla and cinnamon. Soak each slice of bread in egg mixture. Spray pan with cooking spray. Place toast in pan and cook for 2 minutes per side, serve hot with real maple syrup or fresh fruit.

Granola

Prep Time: 30 Minutes   **Baking Time:** 10-15 Minutes

4 cup rolled oats
1 cup wheat bran
1 cup wheat germ
1 cup sesame seeds
1 cup sunflower seeds
1 cup cashews
1 cup almonds
1 cup walnuts
1 cup pecans
½ cup canola oil
½ cup honey
2 teaspoon vanilla extract
½ cup unsweetened coconut
1 cup raisins
1 teaspoon salt

Mix in large bowl and spread a thin layer on cookie sheet. Cook at 350° until golden brown, about 10 to 15 minutes.

Pancakes

Prep Time: 10 Minutes **Cooking Time:** 4 minutes
Servings: 6-8

1 cup whole wheat flour
2 teaspoon baking powder
½ teaspoon salt
1 tablespoon honey
1 egg white
1 cup skim milk
2 tablespoon canola oil

Stir together dry ingredients in a medium mixing bowl, make a well in the center and set aside. In another bowl combine the egg white, milk, honey, and oil, mix. Add egg mixture to dry ingredients, stir just until moist. Pour about ¼ cup batter onto a hot, lightly sprayed skillet. Cook over medium heat for 2 minutes per side. Serve warm with real maple syrup or fresh fruit.

Waffles

Prep Time: 15 Minutes   **Cooking Time:** 5 Minutes
Servings: 5-6

1½ cup whole wheat flour
2 teaspoon baking powder
½ teaspoon salt
1½ tablespoon honey
2 egg whites
1 cup skim milk
2 tablespoon canola oil

Combine egg whites, milk and oil. Mix in dry ingredients. Stir only until batter is smooth. Bake in hot waffle grill.

Chapter 14
Main Course

- Apple Chicken
- Barbecue Chicken
- Blackened Halibut
- Broiled Salmon
- Buffalo Tacos
- Cashew Chicken Stir Fry
- Chicken Enchiladas
- Chicken Fajitas
- Chicken Spaghetti
- Citrus Salmon
- Crab Enchiladas
- Crispy Baked Chicken
- Crock Pot Stew
- Curry Salmon
- Easy Sloppy Joes
- Foil Cooked Salmon
- Grilled Dill Salmon
- Grilled Salmon
- Ginger Almond Chicken Stir Fry
- Grandma's Lemon Grilled Chicken
- Grilled Cajun Fish
- Herbed Chicken
- Herb Basted Salmon
- Herb Salmon Fillets
- Honey Baked Chicken
- Italian Chicken
- Kick It Up Fish
- Lasagna
- Lemon Pepper Halibut
- Marinated Chicken Breasts
- Marinara Sauce
- Marinated Salmon
- Meatloaf
- Meat Roll
- Mexican Plate
- Mexican Turkey Burger
- Mushroom Tarragon Fish
- Mustard Salmon
- Oriental Chicken Tenders
- Oven Fried Fish
- Ratatouille with Fettuccini
- Salmon Patties
- Salmon and Zucchini
- Soft Chicken Tacos
- Southwest Chicken
- Spaghetti Sauce
- Spicy Chicken Breasts
- Spicy Oven Fried Chicken
- Stuffed Bell Peppers
- Szechwan Buffalo Stir Fry
- Teriyaki Halibut
- Teriyaki Salmon
- Turkey and Broccoli Lasagna
- Vegetable Marinara Sauce with Pasta

Apple Chicken

Prep Time: 15 Minutes   **Cooking Time:** 20 Minutes
Servings: 6

6 chicken breasts,
1 cup unsweetened apple juice
¼ teaspoon ground ginger
1 tablespoon cornstarch
2 cup pink lady apples, chopped
2 stalks celery, sliced
3 tablespoon raisins
1 tablespoon sliced green onion
1 tablespoon lemon juice
¼ teaspoon salt

Place chicken, ½ cup apple juice, and lemon juice, salt and pepper in skillet sprayed with Pam. Heat to boiling, cover and simmer for 20 minutes or until chicken is tender and done. Remove chicken. Mix remaining apple juice and cornstarch. Stirring constantly. Add remaining ingredients. Arrange chicken on plate. Top with apple mixture.

Barbecue Chicken

Prep Time: 20 Minutes **Baking Time:** 60 Minutes
Servings: 3-4

3 chicken breasts
1/3 cup vinegar
¼ cup canola oil
1 teaspoon Worcestershire sauce
½ cup tomato sauce
½ teaspoon dry mustard
½ teaspoon grated onion
1 clove garlic, minced
¾ teaspoon salt
¼ teaspoon paprika
Few drops of Tabasco sauce

Cut chicken into serving pieces. Brush lightly with oil. Sprinkle with salt and pepper. Arrange pieces in open roasting pan so that they do not overlap. Bake in 475° oven for 20 minutes, turning pieces after 10 minutes. Combine all other ingredients and mix well, pour over chicken. Reduce heat and bake 45 minutes, basting occasionally.

Blackened Halibut

Prep Time: 15 Minutes   **Cooking Time:** 5 Minutes
Servings: 4

4 pieces of halibut, filleted
¼ cup Melted Benecol
1 tablespoon paprika
2½ teaspoon salt
1 teaspoon onion powder
1 teaspoon red pepper
1 teaspoon garlic powder
¾ teaspoon white pepper
¾ teaspoon black pepper
½ teaspoon dry thyme
½ teaspoon oregano

Dip fish in melted benecol and then in mixture of seasonings. Cook on George Foreman Grill (450°) or in skillet, preheated until pan is very hot, spray with Pam just prior to cooking. On grill, cook for 4 minutes. In skillet cook 2 minutes on one side, turn and cook for another minute.

Broiled Salmon

Prep Time: 10 Minutes   **Broiling Time:** 10 Minutes
Servings: 2

2 salmon steaks
½ cup olive oil
¼ cup soy sauce
½ teaspoon dried dill weed
2 tablespoon lemon juice
½ tablespoon ground cloves

Prepare a sauce of the olive oil, soy sauce, dill weed, lemon juice and cloves. Mix well and brush over salmon steaks. Place on baking sheet. Broil salmon for about 5 minutes on both sides until lightly browned and tender. Do not overcook. Baste as needed.

Buffalo Tacos

Prep Time: 30 Minutes   **Cooking Time:** 20 Minutes
Servings: 6

1 pound ground buffalo
1 large onion chopped
1 teaspoon salt
½ teaspoon pepper
1 tablespoon chili powder
2 teaspoon cumin
1 glove garlic, minced
¼ cup water
1 can fat free refried beans
2 tomatoes, chopped
2 cup lettuce, shredded
8 whole wheat tortilla shells
salsa
guacamole

Brown meat with ½ the onion, until meat is brown and onion is tender, add spices and water. Simmer for 20 minutes and prepare tacos with remaining ingredients. Warm shells in microwave for approximately 15 seconds each.

Cashew Chicken Stir Fry

Prep Time: 20 Minutes   **Cooking Time:** 10 Minutes
Servings: 4

2 cup cubed chicken, about 2 breasts
2 tablespoon canola oil
2 cloves garlic (minced)
2 tablespoon fresh ginger
1 cup Chinese pea pods
1 cup bamboo shoots
1 cup sliced water chestnuts
2 cup fresh mushrooms, sliced
¾ cup diagonally cut celery
½ cup chopped green onion
¾ cup chicken broth
1 teaspoon salt
2 tablespoon cornstarch
¼ cup water
1 tablespoon soy sauce
1 cup toasted cashew nuts

In small bowl combine broth, salt, cornstarch, water, and soy sauce, set aside. Heat wok on high. Put oil, garlic and ginger in pan heat for 1 minute to mix flavors. Add chicken cook for 3-5 minutes. Remove chicken from pan and set aside. Put vegetables in wok and cook, add nuts, chicken and sauce, cook for 2-3 minutes until sauce thickens. Serve hot.

Chicken Enchiladas

Prep Time: 30 Minutes   **Baking Time:** 35-40 Minutes
Servings: 8

1 med. onion, chopped and sautéed in Benecol
8 oz. fat free cream cheese, softened
1 can green chilies, chopped
8 whole wheat flour tortillas
2 cups salsa
8 oz. fat free sour cream
1 cup fat free cheddar cheese, shredded

Combine chicken, onion, cream cheese and chilies. Spoon into tortilla and roll up. Place in greased baking dish seam side down. Combine salsa and sour cream. Pour over top of tortillas. Bake in preheated 350° oven for 35 to 40 minutes. Sprinkle with cheese and return to oven until cheese is melted.

Chicken Fajitas

Prep Time: 30 Minutes   **Marinade** 45 Minutes
Cooking Time: 7 Minutes   **Servings:** 4

2/3 cup canola oil
1/3 cup lime juice
2 tablespoon chopped green chilies
2 cloves garlic, chopped
2 chicken breasts (sliced)
1 red bell pepper
1 green bell pepper
1 onion sliced
4 whole wheat tortillas

In a baking pan, stir together all marinade ingredients. Add chicken and vegetables. Marinade for at least 45 minutes in the refrigerator. Remove from marinade and drain. Grill chicken and vegetables on George Forman Grill at 375° for 7 minutes or broil in oven for 7 minutes, stirring a couple of times. Serve with salsa, guacamole, and fat free cheese.

Chicken Spaghetti

Prep Time: 30 Minutes   **Cooking Time:** 35-40 Minutes
Servings: 6

¼ cup canola oil
3 chicken breasts, cut up into pieces
1 onion, chopped
2 cloves garlic, chopped
½ cup water
1 can tomato paste
1-2 cup water
1 cup whole wheat flour
Salt & pepper

Put oil in a large pot. Salt and pepper the chicken then add chicken to large pot. Cook over medium heat until chicken is brown on all sides. Sauté chopped onions and garlic then add to chicken in pot. Using skillet, put ½ cup water, add salt and pepper and flour. Make a dark roux. Add tomato paste to your roux. Stir well. Add about 2 cup or more water to the roux to make your gravy. Pour gravy over chicken and onions in the large pot. Add more water to thin your gravy to the consistency you like your gravy to be. You may need to add more salt and pepper. Cook chicken in gravy over medium to low heat, stirring occasionally for 30 to 45 minutes. Serve over hot whole wheat spaghetti.

Citrus Salmon

Prep Time: 20 Minutes   **Marinade:** 3 Hours
Broiling Time: 8 Minutes   **Servings:** 4

4 salmon fillets or steaks
½ teaspoon each orange, lemon & lime zest
½ cup fresh orange juice
2 tablespoon lemon
2 tablespoon lime juice
¼ cup onion, minced
1 tablespoon honey
½ tablespoon hot red chili pepper, minced or ¼ teaspoon red pepper flakes (optional)
1 tablespoon Benecol, divided

In a shallow glass or ceramic dish arrange salmon steaks in a single layer. In a small bowl combine the orange, lemon and lime zest, juices, onion, honey and pepper. Mix well; pour over salmon, cover and refrigerate. Marinate fish, turning occasionally, for at least 3 hours. Melt Benecol. Transfer salmon to broiler rack, and reserve marinade. Brush steaks with melted Benecol and broil 2 inches from heat, 4 minutes on each side. Marinade as desired.

Crab Enchiladas

Prep Time: 35 minutes **Baking Time:** 40 Minutes
Servings 4

1 package imitation crab meat
12 corn tortillas
1 red onion, finely chopped
3 cloves garlic, minced
1 teaspoon cumin
1 teaspoon pepper
2 tablespoon olive oil
1/3 tablespoon whole wheat flour
1½ cup fat free sour cream
1 can chicken broth
1 tablespoon jalapeno peppers, chopped
2 cans green chilies
2 tablespoon cilantro
1½ cup fat free shredded mozzarella cheese

Prepare baking dish by spraying bottom and sides of pan with cooking spray, set aside for later. Flake fis and put it in a mixing bowl and set aside. Wrap tortillas in foil and heat in oven at 350° for 10-15 minutes. In medium sauce pan cook red onion, garlic, cumin, and pepper in olive oil until onions are tender. Add flour to sour cream and mix well, add sour cream, broth, and peppers to onion mixture. Stir over medium heat until mixture begins to thicken. Add half of the cheese and mix. Add ¾ cup of sour cream mixture and the cilantro to fish and mix until combined. Scoop about ¼ cup of fish mixture into each tortilla and roll, place in baking dish seam side down. Top with remaining sour cream sauce. Bake covered at 350° for 30-35 minutes, add remaining cheese and return to oven for 5 more minutes to melt cheese. Allow to stand for 10 minutes before serving.

Crispy Baked Chicken

Prep Time: 15 Minutes **Cooking Time:** 60 Minutes
Servings: 4

2 tablespoon fat free mayonnaise
2 tablespoon prepared mustard
¼ cup wheat germ
1/3 cup fine dry whole wheat bread crumbs
½ teaspoon ground thyme
¼ teaspoon salt
4 chicken breast halves
cooking spray

Combine mayonnaise and mustard in a small bowl; stir well. Combine wheat germ and spices in a shallow bowl. Brush each chicken breast with mustard mixture, dredge in bread crumb mixture. Place chicken in a baking dish that has been coated with cooking spray. Cover and bake at 350° for 40 minutes. Uncover and bake an additional 20 minutes or until chicken is tender.

Crock Pot Stew

**Prep Time: 30 Minutes   Cooking Time: 6 Hours
Servings: 6-8**

3 carrots, sliced
1 onion, chopped
1 cup mushrooms, sliced
1 cup dry barley
3 pounds buffalo roast cubes
¼ cup whole wheat flour
2 cup water
2 teaspoon worchestershire sauce
1 bay leaf
1 tablespoon salt
1 teaspoon pepper

Toss buffalo cubes in flour. Put all ingredients in crock pot and cook on high for about 6 hours.

Curry Salmon

Prep Time: 15 Minutes   **Cooking Time:** 6 Minutes
Servings: 2

2 salmon steaks or fillets
1 tablespoon red wine vinegar
2 tablespoon Benecol, melted
2 teaspoon whole wheat flour
1 teaspoon dried snipped chives
1 teaspoon curry powder
1/8 teaspoon salt
½ cup skim milk
2 tablespoon peanuts, chopped

Sprinkle vinegar over salmon and microwave at 100% covered, 3 to 6 minutes, turning over halfway through cooking time. In a small sauce pan, melt Benecol; stir in dry ingredients, add milk and simmer 1 to 2 minutes until thick. Spoon over steaks and add peanuts. Makes 2 servings.

Easy Sloppy Joes

Prep Time: 20 Minutes **Simmer Time:** 20 Minutes
Servings: 8

1 pound ground buffalo or turkey
1 onion
1 teaspoon salt
½ teaspoon pepper
1 glove garlic, minced
1 tablespoon vinegar
1 tablespoon dry mustard
1 can tomato sauce
¼ cup honey
8 whole wheat buns

Brown meat and onion until crumbled and onions are clear and tender, and remaining ingredients and simmer for 20 minutes. Serve on whole wheat buns.

Foil Cooked Salmon
Prep Time: 10 Minutes   Cooking Time: 12 Minutes
Servings: 4

4 Fresh salmon fillets or steaks
1 teaspoon season salt
1 onion, minced
¼ cup dill leaves, chopped
¼ cup fresh rosemary, chopped
¼ cup fresh parsley, chopped
2 tablespoon Lemon juice
2 tablespoon Benecol

Salt and pepper salmon steaks (individually wrapped in foil). Sprinkle with season salt, onion, dill, rosemary and parsley. Sprinkle lemon juice and top with a little Benecol. Wrap/seal in foil (make sure ends are sealed loosely). Put on BBQ grate, about 10-12 minutes. Do not overcook. When fish flakes, remove to eat.

Grilled Dill Salmon

Prep Time: 15 Minutes **Cooking Time:** 12 Minutes
Servings: 4

½ teaspoon lemon zest
1 cup plain nonfat yogurt
¼ cup sliced green onions
¼ cup snipped fresh dill or 1 teaspoon dried dill weed
1 tablespoon capers
4 salmon fillets, skinned
1 tablespoon olive oil
Brown rice
Lemon slices

In a small mixing bowl, combine lemon zest, yogurt, green onions, dill and capers. Add half the mixture to the blender container; cover and blend until smooth. Stir into remaining mixture in the bowl. Brush salmon fillets with olive oil. Spray grill rack with non-stick spray coating. Grill salmon over medium-hot heat for 5 minutes. Turn salmon. Grill 5 to 7 minutes more until fish just flakes with a fork. Top salmon with 2 tablespoon of sauce. Serve with brown rice and grilled lemon slices. Slices of lemon may be grilled by adding lemon slices to the grill when you turn the fish.

Grilled Salmon

Prep Time: 10 Minutes Marinade: 1 Hour
Grilling Time: 12 Minutes Servings: 6

6 salmon steaks, 3/4 inch thick
½ cup white wine vinegar
¼ cup canola oil
2 tablespoon chives, chopped
1 teaspoon leaf thyme, crumbled
1 teaspoon salt
¼ teaspoon freshly ground black pepper

Combine all ingredients except salmon to make marinade. Place steaks in a large glass dish and pour marinade over all; cover with plastic wrap. Marinate at room temperature for 1 hour. Grill over medium fire, 4 inches from heat, turning and basting with marinade, for 12 to 15 minutes, or until fish flakes easily with a fork.

Ginger Almond Chicken Stir Fry

Prep Time: 30 Minutes   Cooking Time: 15 Minutes
Servings: 4

2 teaspoon slivered almonds
2 chicken breasts, diced into ½ inch cubes
½ green pepper, cut into ½ inch strips
4-5 stalks celery and tops, sliced diagonally
3 green onions and tops, sliced
½ cup fresh snow peas
2 tablespoon canola oil
1 teaspoon salt
1 teaspoon ginger
½ teaspoon pepper
1/8 teaspoon garlic powder
1 chicken bouillon cube dissolved in 1 cup boiling water
1 tablespoon cornstarch dissolved in ¼ cup cold water
1 tablespoon soy sauce
1 tablespoon lemon juice

Stir fry chicken in hot oil. Add salt, ginger, pepper and nuts and stir fry for about 5-6 minutes. Spoon from pan and keep warm. Add celery, pepper, and onions to hot oil in pan. Stir constantly several minutes or until desired doneness. Add pea pods and stir 1 minute more. Re-add chicken mixture to pan with vegetables. Add bouillon with soy sauce and lemon juice, cook until bubbly. Turn heat down and add cornstarch mixture and stir until thickened and clear.

Grandma's Lemon Grilled Chicken
Prep Time: 10 Minutes   Marinade: Overnight
Cooking Time: 10 Minutes   Servings: 4

½ cup canola oil
¼ cup water
1 tablespoon onion (minced)
½ cup lemon juice
½ teaspoon salt
½ teaspoon paprika
½ teaspoon pepper
4 chicken breasts

Blend together oil, water, onion, lemon juice, and spices. Marinade chicken in sauce for several hours or overnight, drain chicken, reserve marinade. Broil chicken in oven; use George Foreman grill or barbecue grill. Baste with marinade throughout cooking. For George Foreman Grill cook at 350° for 7 minutes. On grill or in oven, cook for 5 minutes per side.

Grilled Cajun Fish

Prep Time: 15 Minutes   **Cooking Time:** 8-12 minutes
Servings: 4

4 pieces of halibut
1 tablespoon lime juice
1 teaspoon white pepper
1 teaspoon garlic powder
½ teaspoon cayenne pepper
1 teaspoon onion powder
1 teaspoon paprika
1 teaspoon black pepper

Combine seasonings in a small bowl. Brush halibut with lime juice and sprinkle/rub with seasoning. Allow to sit for 10 minutes. If using a George Foreman grill cook it at 375° for 7 minutes. You can also broil it or grill it. If grilling use a medium heat for 5 minutes per side. Broiling it generally takes 4-7 minutes per side.

Herbed Chicken

Prep Time: 25 Minutes **Cooking Time:** 40 Minutes
Servings: 4

1 tablespoon olive oil
1 medium onion, chopped
1 red pepper, chopped
6 fresh mushrooms, thinly sliced
1/3 cup chicken broth
2 tablespoon red wine vinegar
1 can tomato sauce
2 garlic cloves, minced
1 teaspoon honey
¼ teaspoon salt
¼ teaspoon pepper
3 chicken breasts, cut into chunks
2 tablespoon chopped fresh basil or 1 teaspoon dried basil
1 tablespoon chopped fresh sage or ½ teaspoon dried sage
1 pound. dry whole wheat linguine or spaghetti, cooked and drained

In a skillet, heat oil over medium high. Sauté onion, peppers and mushrooms until tender. Add broth and vinegar; bring to a boil. Boil 2 minutes. Add tomato sauce, garlic, honey, salt and pepper. Bring to a boil. Reduce heat; cover and simmer 25 minutes. Add chicken, basil and sage. Cook, uncovered, 15 minutes more or until chicken is done and sauce is lightly thickened. Serve chicken and sauce over pasta.

Herb Basted Salmon

Prep Time: 15 Minutes   **Cooking Time:** 6 Minutes
Servings: 4

2 tablespoon olive oil
2 tablespoon melted Benecol
1 tablespoon fresh chopped basil
1 tablespoon fresh chopped parsley
1 teaspoon grated lemon peel
Salt and pepper to taste
4 salmon steaks or salmon fillet

Combine all ingredients except salmon. Baste salmon with mixture, cooking according to desired methods. Broil 4 to 6 inches from heat, 10 minutes. Brush with baste as needed.

Herb Salmon Fillets

Prep Time: 20 Minutes   **Broiling Time:** 10 Minutes
Servings: 6

6 salmon steaks
½ cup virgin olive oil
¼ cup chopped dill
½ cup olive oil
3 tablespoon wine vinegar
1 tablespoon imported mustard
1 clove garlic
½ cup Italian parsley
½ cup green onions
¼ cup chives, chopped
¼ cup fresh dill

Arrange filets on broiler pan evenly. Brush olive oil over each filet. Sprinkle chopped dill over each filet. Lightly salt and pepper to taste. Broil for 5 minutes per side, check to see if pieces are cooked through. Blend remaining ingredients in food processor or blender until herbs are finely chopped. Do not overblend, as mixture should have texture. Serve as sauce with salmon filets.

Honey Baked Chicken

Prep Time: 15 Minutes **Baking Time:** 1¼ Hour
Servings: 6-8

3 or 4 pounds chicken, cut up
½ cup smart balance, melted
½ cup honey
1 teaspoon salt
¼ cup mustard
1 teaspoon curry

Combine smart balance, honey, salt, mustard and curry. Pour over chicken. Bake at 350° for 1¼ hours. Basting every 15 minutes.

Italian Chicken

Prep Time: 15 Minutes **Baking Time:** 1 Hour
Servings: 4

4 chicken breast
cooking spray
2-3 cloves garlic, minced
Sage leaves, crumpled
Parsley
Garlic salt
Oregano
Salt
Pepper

Prepare baking sheet with cooking spray. Place chicken on baking sheet, spray chicken with cooking spray. Spread garlic over chicken pieces. Sprinkle other seasonings over chicken. Bake at 350° for 1 hour.

Kick It Up Fish

Prep Time: 15 Minutes   **Cooking Time:** 8-12 Minutes
Servings: 4

4 pieces of halibut or orange roughy
1 cup milk
¼ cup apple cider vinegar
1 tablespoon onion powder
1 teaspoon cumin
1 tablespoon dry mustard
½ teaspoon allspice
½ teaspoon garlic powder
½ teaspoon cayenne pepper

In a shallow bowl combine milk and vinegar, place fish in bowl and turn to coat. Allow to soak for 30 minutes. Meanwhile combine spices in a shallow bowl. Drain fish, and dredge in spices. If using a George Foreman grill cook it at 375° for 7 minutes. You can also broil it or grill it. If grilling use a medium heat for 5 minutes per side. Broiling it generally takes 4-7 minutes per side.

Lasagna

Prep Time: 1½ Hours **Cooking Time:** 40-45 Minutes
Servings: 8

2 pounds ground buffalo or turkey
1 onion, chopped
2 cloves garlic, minced
2 cans diced tomatoes
1 can tomato paste
2 cans tomato sauce
1 teaspoon salt
1 teaspoon pepper
1 bay leaf
2 teaspoon basil
2 teaspoon oregano
1 teaspoon marjoram
½ teaspoon rosemary
1 package whole wheat lasagna noodles
2 cup fat free cottage cheese
2 cup fat free sour cream
½ cup fresh chives
1 package fat free grated mozzarella cheese

In pot cook meat, onion and garlic until meat is browned. Add the tomato products, salt, pepper and the bay leaf. Allow to simmer for up to 3 hours (at least one hour, longer is better). Add remaining spices except chives. Allow to cook an additional 10 minutes. Meanwhile prepare noodles as directed on package (al dante, or until firm), drain and rinse (I usually lay out on a tea towel to absorb the extra moisture). In a mixing bowl combine cottage cheese, sour cream and chives, set aside. Now you begin to layer. Lightly spray a baking pan (9 X 13). Put a thin layer of the meat sauce on the bottom to ensure it will not stick. Next layer noodles laying side by side, spread approximately 1/3 of the sour cream mixture and then 1/3 of the meat sauce, sprinkle with cheese, (use a little if you don't like cheese more if you do). Layer with noodles next and repeat as above, for a total of 3 layers. Bake at 375° for 40-45 minutes. Allow to stand for 10 minutes prior to serving.

Lemon Pepper Halibut

Prep Time: 15 minutes   **Cooking Time:** 8-12 Minutes
Servings: 4

4 pieces of halibut
2 tablespoon lemon juice
1 tablespoon black pepper
2 teaspoon lemon zest
1 teaspoon coriander
1 teaspoon onion powder
1 teaspoon thyme

Combine spices and lemon zest. Brush halibut with lemon juice, and sprinkle with spices. Allow flavors to blend for 10 minutes. If using a George Foreman grill cook it at 375° for 7 minutes. You can also broil it or grill it. If grilling use a medium heat for 5 minutes per side. Broiling it generally takes 4-7 minutes per side. This recipe also works well for chicken.

Marinated Chicken Breasts

Prep Time: 20 Minutes **Marinade:** Overnight
Cooking Time: 10 Minutes **Servings** 6

6 chicken breasts
3 cloves garlic, crushed
1½ teaspoon salt
½ cup molasses
3 tablespoon grainy mustard
¼ cup cider vinegar
Juice of 1 lime
Juice of ½ lemon
6 tablespoon olive oil
Black pepper to taste

Put the chicken breasts in a shallow bowl. Mix garlic, salt, molasses, mustard, vinegar, and lime and lemon juices. Blend well. Whisk in olive oil and add pepper. Pour over the chicken and refrigerate overnight, covered. Turn over. Remove from the refrigerator 1 hour before you want to cook and let come to room temperature. Grill approximately 4 minutes per side or until done. Or Grill on George Foreman Grill for 5-7 minutes at 350°.

Marinara Sauce

Prep Time: 20 Minutes **Cooking Time:** 1 Hour
Servings: 4

1 cup onions, chopped
1 cup bell pepper, chopped
½ cup celery, sliced
2 cloves garlic, minced
2 tablespoon olive oil
2 cans tomatoes, diced
1 can tomato paste
½ cup water
1 teaspoon salt
½ teaspoon pepper
1 teaspoon basil
1 teaspoon oregano
1 teaspoon thyme
1 teaspoon honey
whole wheat pasta

In large pot cook onions, peppers, celery and garlic in hot olive oil until tender. Stir in tomatoes, tomato paste, water, salt and pepper. Bring to a boil reduce heat, cover and let simmer for 45 minutes, stirring often. Add remaining spices and cook an additional 10 minutes. Serve.

Marinated Salmon

Prep Time: 15 Minutes **Marinade:** 30 minutes
Grilling: 8 minutes **Servings:** 4

4 pieces of salmon
½ teaspoon lemon zest
¼ cup fresh lemon juice
1 tablespoon canola oil
1 tablespoon water
1 tablespoon Worcestershire sauce
½ teaspoon rosemary
½ teaspoon thyme
1 clove garlic, minced

In a shallow dish, combine all the ingredients except the fish. Add fish, turn to coat with marinade. Cover and marinade for 30 minutes, turning occasionally. Drain fish. If using a George Foreman grill cook it at 375° for 7 minutes. You can also broil it or grill it. If grilling use a medium heat for 5 minutes per side. Broiling it generally takes 4-7 minutes per side. Baste with marinade.

Meatloaf

Prep Time: 15 Minutes   **Baking Time:** 1 Hour
Servings: 4-6

1½ pounds ground buffalo or turkey
¼ cup egg beaters
¾ cup whole wheat cracker crumbs
1 onion, chopped
½ bell pepper chopped
1 stalk of celery, chopped
1 can tomato sauce
1 teaspoon salt
1 teaspoon pepper
1 tablespoon prepared mustard

In large bowl combine all the ingredients except ½ can of tomato sauce, stir until well blended. Form into a loaf and place in baking dish sprayed with cooking spray. Spread tomato sauce over top of meatloaf Bake at 350° for 45 minutes to an 1 hour. Allow to sit for 5 minutes prior to serving.

Meat Roll

Prep Time: 45 Minutes **Cooking Time:** 75 Minutes
Servings: 8-10

1½ pounds ground buffalo
1 cup whole wheat cracker crumbs
2 teaspoon Worchestershire sauce
1 can chicken broth
½ cup brown rice
1 clove garlic, minced
1 teaspoon salt
½ teaspoon pepper
2 dill pickles, chopped
1 onion, minced
1 tablespoon mustard
1 cup fat free grated cheese
½ cup tomato sauce

Cook rice using ½ can broth for liquid. Combine meat, crackers, Worcestershire sauce, remaining broth, rice, and spices, place on a sheet of plastic wrap or foil, shape into a 8X12 inch rectangle. Spread mustard on meat mixture and sprinkle with onions, pickles, and cheese, sprinkle with salt and pepper. Roll lengthwise and place in 9x13 pan. Pour tomato sauce over and bake at 350° for 75 minutes. Slice and serve.

Mexican Plate

Prep Time: 30 Minutes   Servings: 4

1 pound ground turkey
1 tablespoon chili powder
2 teaspoon cumin
2 teaspoon onion powder
1 clove garlic, minced
¼ cup water
baked blue corn chips
Lettuce
Fat free grated mozzarella cheese
Fat free grated cheddar cheese
2 ripe tomatoes
1 can black olives, sliced
1 onion, chopped
1 can black beans
1½ cup egg beaters, scrambled with salt and pepper
Guacamole
Salsa

In skillet brown turkey, add chili powder, cumin, onion powder, garlic and water, simmer for 10 minutes. Put in serving bowl. Set bowls with each of the items on the table. Allow each person to create a unique Mexican plate from the above choices.

Mexican Turkey Burger

Prep Time: 30 Minutes   **Cooking Time:** 8-15 Minutes
Servings: 4

1 pound ground turkey
Bottled mild salsa
½ pound mushrooms
1 tablespoon salad oil
½ teaspoon salt
2 tablespoon fat free mayonnaise
4 whole wheat hamburger buns

In bowl, mix ground turkey and 1/4 cup salsa; shape into 4 patties. Broil or grill until they lose their pink color turning once. Meanwhile, slice mushrooms. In skillet over medium heat, in hot canola oil, cook mushrooms and salt until lightly browned, stirring frequently. In small bowl mix mayonnaise and 1/3 cup salsa. To serve, cut each bun in half. Spread mayonnaise mixture on bottom halves of buns. Top with turkey patties and mushrooms.

Mushroom Tarragon Fish

Prep Time: 20 Minutes   **Baking Time:** 12 Minutes
Servings: 4

4 pieces of halibut or salmon
salt and pepper
2 tablespoon olive oil
2 cup fresh mushrooms, sliced
½ cup green onions, sliced
½ teaspoon tarragon
½ teaspoon thyme

Spray baking dish with cooking spray, place fish in baking dish, and salt and pepper. Heat olive oil in saucepan, and mushrooms, onions, and spices. Cook until mushrooms are tender. Spoon mushroom mixture over fish. Bake covered at 450° for 12 to 18 minutes.

Mustard Salmon

Prep Time: 15 Minutes **Broiling Time:** 12 Minutes
Servings: 4

4 salmon fillets
2 tablespoon Dijon mustard
1 tablespoon olive oil
1 tablespoon honey
1 teaspoon grated lemon peel
1 T. lemon juice
Parsley sprigs
Lemon wedges
Salt & pepper

Rinse salmon fillets and pat dry. Place fillets, skin side down, on a piece of heavy-duty foil set in a rimmed 10 x 15 inch pan. Mix the mustard, oil, honey, lemon peel and lemon juice. Brush fish with all of the mustard mixture. Broil fish about 5 inches from heat just until it looks slightly translucent and wet in thickest part (cut to test), 9-12 minutes. Lift foil to transfer fillet to a serving platter. Garnish with parsley and lemon wedges. Add salt and pepper to taste.

Oriental Chicken Tenders

Prep Time: 10 Minutes **Marinade:** Overnight
Cooking Time: 20 Minutes **Servings:** 4-6

1 cup soy sauce
1/3 cup honey
4 teaspoon canola oil
1½ teaspoon ground ginger
1 teaspoon five spice powder (available in Chinese markets)
2 bunches green onion
4 chicken breast cut into strips

Blend soy sauce, honey, oil, ginger and five spice powder in a large bowl until the honey dissolves. Stir in green onions. Add chicken tenders to marinade. Turn to coat. Cover chicken and refrigerate overnight. Preheat oven to 350° Drain chicken RESERVING MARINADE. Arrange chicken in dish and bake for 20-30 minutes until brown and tender, while basting occasionally with marinade.

Oven Fried Fish

Prep Time: 10 Minutes **Baking Time:** 8-12 minutes
Servings: 4

4 pieces of halibut
½ cup whole wheat bread crumbs
2 tablespoon cornmeal
2 tablespoon pecans (finely chopped)
¼ teaspoon salt
½ teaspoon pepper
¼ cup whole wheat flour
¼ cup skim milk

Prepare a baking pan by spraying with cooking spray. In a shallow bowl mix bread crumbs, cornmeal, pecans, salt and pepper. Coat each piece of fish with the flour, dip in milk and then coat with crumb mixture. Spray fish with cooking spray and arrange in one layer in baking pan. Bake at 375° for 8-12 minutes.

Ratatouille with Fettuccini

Prep Time: 30 Minutes   **Cooking Time:** 10 Minutes
Servings: 8

1 tablespoon extra virgin olive oil
2 cloves fresh garlic
1 cup onion, chopped
1 eggplant, diced, skin on
3 zucchinis, diced
2 yellow squash, diced
1 red pepper, diced
1 green pepper, diced
2 cup mushrooms, sliced
5 tomatoes, peeled, seeded & chopped
1 tablespoon fresh oregano
1 tablespoon fresh basil
Salt & pepper to taste
1 pound whole wheat Fettuccini

Prepare Fettuccini according to package directions. Heat oil in large pan, add garlic and onion; cook until tender. Add all vegetables and stir well. Let simmer for about 5 minutes. Do not over cook vegetables. Add fresh spices and salt and pepper to taste. Serve over Fettuccini.

Salmon Patties

Prep Time: 25 Minutes **Cooking Time:** 10 minutes
Servings: 4

½ cup egg beaters
2 tablespoon skim milk
1 small onion, chopped
½ green pepper, chopped
2 cans boneless, skinless salmon, drained
¾ cup whole wheat crackers (crushed)
1 clove garlic, minced
1 tablespoon lemon juice
½ teaspoon salt
½ teaspoon pepper

Prepare a baking pan by spraying bottom with cooking spray. Combine all the ingredients, mix well. Form patties and spray the patties with cooking spray. Bake at 375° for 6-10 minutes or until crispy.

Salmon and Zucchini

Prep Time: 20 Minutes   **Cooking Time:** 10 minutes
Servings: 4

4 salmon steaks or fillets
½ cup chicken broth
3 zucchinis, sliced
¼ teaspoon salt
¾ teaspoon fresh basil, minced
½ cup skim milk

Place salmon in large saucepan or skillet that has been coated with cooking spray. Add milk and broth. Cover and bring to a boil; reduce heat and simmer until fish is done, about 6 minutes. Cut zucchini into small strips; steam with a vegetable steamer for two to three minutes. Pour into a bowl and toss gently with basil. Transfer to serving plates. Top with salmon. Garnish with basil.

Soft Chicken Tacos

Prep Time: 15 Minutes **Cooking Time:** 20 Minutes
Servings: 10

10 whole wheat flour tortillas
4 chicken breasts (cut in ¼ inch strips)
½ cup chopped onion
1 can tomato sauce
1 teaspoon garlic salt
½ teaspoon salt
2 teaspoon ground cumin
1 tablespoon chili powder
1 teaspoon pepper
Shredded fat free cheese, chopped tomatoes, shredded lettuce, black olives, salsa

In skillet, quickly cook chicken slices and onion, until chicken is done and onion is tender. Add tomato sauce, and spices. Reduce heat and simmer, covered for 15-20 minutes. To serve, place hot meat mixture on heated tortillas and top with choice of fillings. Roll up burrito style. Filling: shredded fat free cheese, chopped tomatoes, shredded lettuce, sliced pitted ripe olives, and salsa.

Southwest Chicken

Prep Time: 15 Minutes **Marinade:** 1 Hour
Grilling: 8-12 Minutes **Servings:** 4

Juice of 3 limes
¼ cup soy sauce
1½ teaspoon olive oil
1 tablespoon chili powder
1½ teaspoon cumin
1½ teaspoon coriander
6 cloves garlic, minced
1½ teaspoon honey
2 whole chicken breasts
¼ cup rice wine vinegar

Combine all the ingredients except the chicken and vinegar in a shallow bowl. Lay chicken in bowl and turn to coat. Marinade for at least 1 hour. Add vinegar just prior to cooking. Remove from marinade. Grill approximately 4 minutes per side or until done. Or Grill on George Foreman Grill for 5-7 minutes at 350°. Baste as desired with marinade.

Spaghetti Sauce

Prep Time: 25 Minutes **Cooking Time:** 2 Hours
Servings: 4-6

1 pound ground buffalo or turkey
1 onion, chopped
1 bell pepper, chopped
2 stalks celery, chopped
2 cloves garlic, minced
2 cans tomatoes, whole or diced
1 6 oz can tomato paste
2 8 oz cans tomato sauce
1 tablespoon fresh basil
1 tablespoon fresh oregano
½ teaspoon dried marjoram
1 teaspoon honey
½ teaspoon salt
½ teaspoon pepper
whole wheat pasta

In large pot brown meat with onions, peppers, celery and garlic until meat is browned. Stir in tomatoes, paste and sauce. Bring to a boil and reduce heat. Allow to simmer for 1½. Add remaining spices and cook an additional ½ hour. Meanwhile prepare the pasta as directed on package.

Spicy Chicken Breasts

Prep Time: 10 Minutes **Baking Time:** 1 hour
Servings: 4

4 chicken breasts
2 teaspoon lemon juice
½ teaspoon dry mustard
½ cup skim milk
1 cup non-fat plain yogurt
3 tablespoon soy sauce

Arrange chicken in baking dish. Combine lemon juice, mustard, mayonnaise, yogurt, and soy sauce in small bowl, spoon over chicken. Bake uncovered at 350° for 60 minutes or until chicken is golden. Arrange chicken on platter, put leftover sauce blender. Cover and blend until smooth, pour over chicken.

Spicy Oven Fried Chicken

Prep Time: 30 Minutes   **Baking Time:** 55 Minutes
Servings: 6

6 chicken breasts
½ cup cornmeal
½ cup whole wheat flour
1½ teaspoon salt
1½ teaspoon chili powder
½ teaspoon oregano
¼ teaspoon pepper
2-3 chicken breasts
½ cup skim milk
cooking spray

Prepare baking pan with Pam spray. Combine dry ingredients. Wash chicken and pat dry with paper towel. Dip chicken in milk; coat with cornmeal mixture. Place in baking pan, spray with cooking spray. Bake at 375° for 50-55 minutes.

Stuffed Bell Peppers

Prep Time: 30 Minutes **Baking Time:** 45 Minutes
Servings: 4

½ cup barley
1 cup water
4 bell pepper, generally equal in size
1 pound ground buffalo or turkey
¼ cup egg beaters
1 onion, chopped
1 stalk of celery, chopped
½ tablespoon Worcestershire sauce
½ teaspoon basil
½ teaspoon oregano
1 can tomato sauce
½ teaspoon salt
½ teaspoon pepper

In small saucepan cook barley with water for 1-12 minutes or until tender. Prepare bell peppers, by cutting off the tops and cleaning out the veins and seeds, set aside. Combine the barley with the remaining ingredients except ½ can of tomato sauce. Blend well. Stuff peppers with meat mixture. Place in lightly sprayed baking dish. Pour remaining tomato sauce on top and bake at 350° for 45 minutes.

Szechwan Buffalo Stir Fry

Prep Time: 20 Minutes   **Cooking Time:** 10 Minutes
Servings: 4

1 pound buffalo steak, thinly sliced
3 tablespoon rice wine vinegar
3 tablespoon soy sauce
2 tablespoon water
2 tablespoon hoisin sauce
2 teaspoon cornstarch
1 tablespoon grated ginger root
1 teaspoon honey
1 teaspoon crushed red pepper
½ teaspoon black pepper
2 cloves garlic, minced
1 cup sliced carrots
1 red bell pepper sliced
1½ broccoli, bite size pieces
1 tablespoon canola oil
1 clove garlic, sliced
1 tablespoon ginger root slices
Brown rice

Stir together the vinegar, soy sauce, water, hoisin sauce, cornstarch, ginger, honey, minced garlic, and peppers, set aside. Pour canola oil into wok and heat on high; add sliced garlic and ginger allow to season oil for 1 minute. Remove garlic and ginger and discard. Stir fry carrots in hot oil for about 2 minutes, add the broccoli and bell peppers. Stir fry for an additional 1-2 minutes. Add buffalo stir fry for an additional 2-3 minutes. Stir in sauce (add it to the center of the wok and continue stirring until it is thickened. Serve with brown rice.

Teriyaki Halibut

Prep Time: 20 Minutes **Marinade:** 30 minutes
Cooking: 7-12 minutes **Servings:** 4

4 pieces of halibut
½ cup soy sauce
3 tablespoon orange juice
1 tablespoon canola oil
1 tablespoon fresh ginger root, grated
1 teaspoon honey
1 clove garlic, minced

Combine all ingredients except fish in a shallow bowl to make marinade. Place fish in bowl and turn to coat. Allow to marinade for 30 minutes. Drain fish. If using a George Foreman grill cook it at 375° for 7 minutes. You can also broil it or grill it. If grilling use a medium heat for 5 minutes per side. Broiling it generally takes 4-7 minutes per side. Baste with marinade.

Teriyaki Salmon

Prep Time: 15 Minutes **Marinade:** 2 Hours
Broiling Time: 10 Minutes **Servings:** 4

1 tablespoon fresh ginger root, minced
2 cloves garlic, minced
1 medium onion, finely chopped
2 tablespoon honey
½ cup soy sauce
¼ cup water
4 salmon fillets

Make a sauce from ginger root, garlic, onion, honey, soy sauce and water. Place fish in a single layer in a glass casserole dish. Pour sauce over fish and let marinate 1-2 hours. Preheat broiler. Broil approximately 5 minutes on each side or until flaky. Serve hot with brown rice and mixed vegetables.

Turkey and Broccoli Lasagna

Prep Time: 40 Minutes   **Baking Time:** 40 Minutes
Serving: 6-8

1 package whole wheat lasagna noodles
1 pound ground turkey
1 onion
1 clove garlic, minced
½ teaspoon salt
½ teaspoon pepper
2 cup broccoli, chopped
½ cup water
1 teaspoon thyme
1 cup fat free cottage cheese
1 cup fat free sour cream
¼ cup fresh chives
1 recipe of marinara sauce or 1 bottle of spaghetti sauce (read labels carefully)
2 cup fat free grated mozzarella cheese

Prepare noodles as directed on package (al dante, or until firm), drain and rinse (I usually lay out on a tea towel to absorb the extra moisture). In large skillet cook turkey, onions, garlic, salt and pepper until turkey is browned. Stir in chopped broccoli and water, bring to a boil reduce heat and cook for about 10 minutes add the thyme and cook 2 minutes longer. Drain. In a mixing bowl combine the cottage cheese, sour cream and chives, stir in the turkey mixture. Prepare baking pan (9 X 13) by lightly spraying. Spread a small amount of the marinara sauce and begin layers with the noodles, next the meat and then a layer of marinara, top with cheese, repeat as above, beginning with the noodles for a total of 3 layers. Bake at 375° for 35-40 minutes.

Vegetable Marinara Sauce with Pasta
Prep Time: 30 Minutes   Cooking Time: 30 Minutes
Servings: 10

1 pound ground turkey
2 tablespoon olive oil
1 onion, course chopped
1 bunch fresh green onions, chopped likewise
1 sweet bell pepper, chopped
2 tomato, diced
1 cup fresh spinach, shredded
1 8 oz. can tomato sauce,
1 tablespoon whole wheat flour
1 tablespoon vinegar
1 lemon (juice of)
2 tablespoon soy sauce
2 tablespoon molasses
3 whole bay leaves
1 tablespoon garlic powder
1 tablespoon sweet basil leaves
1 tablespoon oregano leaves
1 teaspoon black pepper
1 dash Tabasco sauce (optional)
1 pound whole wheat pasta

Prepare pasta according to package direction. When pasta finishes cooking, drain and cover with fresh water, place lid on and set aside. In large skillet, brown meat. Remove from skillet. Combine tomato sauce and flour, blend until smooth. Heat olive oil in skillet. Add remaining ingredients, including the meat and cover. Simmer over very low heat for 20 minutes, stirring often. Serve with pasta.

Chapter 15
Vegetables

Baked Beans
Basil and Tomato Penne Pasta
Bean Burritos
Brown Beans (traditional southern dish)
Black Beans and Tomatoes
Cajun Rice
Chili Corn
Citrus Peas
Cowboy Beans
Dilly Zucchini
Easy Baked Beans
Fat Free Fried Rice
Fried Rice
Garlic Broccoli
Green Beans and Almonds
Grilled Corn on The Cob
Hawaiian Fried Rice
Herb Mushrooms
Herbed Tomatoes
Italian Bean Sauté
Italian Carrots
Lemon Broccoli Pasta
Kick It Up Fish
Mozzarella Zucchini
Oriental Broccoli

Oven Fried Zucchini
Roasted Bell Peppers
Red Beans and Rice
Rice Pilaf
Roasted Sweet Potatoes
Sautéed Spinach
Sautéed Spinach and Mushroom
Sautéed Squash
Savory Baked Beans
Savory Asparagus
Spanish Rice
Spicy Black Beans
Spicy Rice
Spicy Tomato Juice
Spicy Zucchini
Sautéed Vegetables
Sweet Pepper Relish
Sweet Rice
Tasty Brown Rice
Vegetable Rice
Vegetable Stir Fry
Vegetable Fried Rice
Vegetable Wrap
Vietnamese Fried Rice
Western Baked Beans

Baked Beans

**Prep Time: 20 Minutes   Cooking Time: 1¼ Hours
Servings: 6**

1 can kidney beans
1 can lima beans
1 can pinto beans
½ can tomato paste
1 large onion, chopped
2 tablespoon apple cider vinegar
2 tablespoon molasses or real maple syrup
2 teaspoon dry mustard
¼ teaspoon cayenne pepper
1 teaspoon salt

Drain part of the liquid off the beans and combine all the ingredients in a baking dish and stir well. Bake covered at 350° for 45 minutes and uncover and bake an additional ½ hour.

Basil and Tomato Penne Pasta

Prep Time: 20 Minutes   Cooking Time: 10 Minutes
Servings: 6-8

1 pound whole wheat penne pasta
8 plum tomatoes
½ cup black olives
1 bunch fresh basil
3 cloves garlic, peeled
1 tablespoon olive oil
1 tablespoon balsamic vinegar
Fresh ground pepper

Wash and dry basil leaves. Place them in a food processor with garlic, olive oil and vinegar. Process until smooth. Cook pasta in boiling water; drain. Add basil mixture to pasta. Stir and keep warm on stove. Slice tomatoes lengthwise. Slice olives. Heat tomatoes and olives together in separate skillet. Cook over medium heat 3 minutes. Toss tomatoes and olives in with pasta mixture. Serve with freshly ground pepper.

Bean Burritos

Prep Time: 20 Minutes   **Baking Time:** 10 Minutes
Servings: 4

2 cans fat free refried beans
1½ cup Fat free grated Cheddar cheese
4 whole wheat flour tortilla shells
1 onion, chopped

In pan, mix beans and onion. Heat until well mixed, add ¾ cup cheese. Fill shells with mixture and put in baking dish, sprinkle remaining cheese on top. Heat at 350° for 10 minutes.

Brown Beans (traditional southern dish)

Prep Time: 30 Minutes   Soaking Time: 6 Hours
Cooking Time: 3 hours   Servings: 8

1 16 oz package of pinto beans
1 16 oz package of turkey bacon
1 teaspoon salt
1 teaspoon pepper
1 can stewed tomatoes
¼ cup chopped jalapeno peppers

Soak beans overnight or for at least 6 hours. Drain and rinse. Put beans in a large pot, add 6 cup water. Chop the bacon into 1 inch pieces and put in pot with beans, add salt and pepper cook over low to medium heat for 2 hours, add the tomatoes and jalapeno peppers, cook an additional hour. Serve with cornbread.

Black Beans and Tomatoes
Prep Time: 20 Minutes   Chilling Time: 2 Hours
Servings: 4

1 can black beans
2 fresh tomatoes
½ cup fresh lemon juice
½ cup fresh parsley
4 to 5 cloves garlic, minced
2 tablespoon olive oil

Rinse and heat black beans. Add olive oil and bring to a slow simmer. Remove from heat and add all ingredients except the lemon juice. Mix thoroughly and refrigerate for 2 hours. Add lemon juice before serving.

Cajun Rice

Prep Time: 15 Minutes **Cooking Time:** 50 Minutes
Servings: 4-6

1 can tomatoes, chopped
½ cup onions, thinly sliced
1 green bell pepper, diced
1 clove garlic, minced
2 tablespoon olive oil
1 cup brown rice
½ teaspoon thyme
½ teaspoon oregano
¾ teaspoon salt
¼ teaspoon pepper
1/8 teaspoon cayenne pepper

Drain tomatoes, reserve liquid. Add enough water to tomato liquid to make 1 1/2 cups. Chop tomatoes reserve. Sauté onions, bell pepper and garlic in olive oil until soft. Add rice, thyme, oregano, salt, pepper and cayenne pepper. Cook stirring, constantly over medium heat; for 1 minute. Add reserved tomatoes and tomato liquid. Bring to a boil. Reduce heat to low cover and cook until all liquid is absorbed, about 50 minutes. Remove from heat and let stand covered for 5 minutes. Uncover and fluff with fork.

Chili Corn

Prep Time: 10 Minutes   Cooking Time: 10 Minutes Servings: 4

2 teaspoon olive oil
2 cloves garlic
1 jalapeno pepper, minced
3 green onions, sliced
1 teaspoon chili powder
½ teaspoon salt
½ teaspoon cumin
4 cup corn
2 tablespoon lime zest

Heat the oil in a large skillet. Add the garlic, jalapenos and onions, cook briefly over low heat. Stir in the spices and cook for about 1 minute. Add the corn and lime zest, cover and cook for another 5 minutes.

Citrus Peas

Prep Time: 10 Minutes **Cooking Time:** 8 Minutes
Servings: 4

2 cup fresh peas
¼ cup green onions, sliced
1 tablespoon fresh mint, chopped
1 teaspoon Benecol
1 teaspoon orange zest
½ teaspoon salt
½ teaspoon garlic powder
¼ teaspoon pepper

Heat 2 cup water until boiling, add peas and cook 3-5 minutes until crisp tender. Drain. Return to pan and add remaining ingredients and heat through.

Cowboy Beans

Prep Time: 30 Minutes   **Cooking Time:** 2 Hours
Servings: 6-8

1¼ cup dried pinto beans
Salt to taste
1 tablespoon canola oil
¾ cup tomatoes, diced
6½ cup water
¾ cup onion, chopped
2 teaspoon jalapenos, chopped and seeded
6 tablespoon chopped fresh coriander

Wash beans well. Put them in a kettle, add the water, bring to a boil partly covered and simmer for 1 hour. Add salt and 1/2 the onion. Continue cooking uncovered 30-45 minutes longer. Heat the oil in a small skillet and add the remaining onions and the Jalapeno peppers. Cook briefly until the onion is wilted. Add the tomatoes and coriander and cook, stirring for 3 more minutes. Scoop out a cup of beans with a little of their liquid, and place in a blender. Blend until smooth. Return this to the beans. Add the tomato mixture to the beans and continue to simmer, about 5 more minutes

Dilly Zucchini

Prep Time: 5 Minutes   **Cooking Time:** 12 Minutes
Servings: 4

2 zucchinis
1 tablespoon Benecol
2 tablespoon fresh dill weed

Cut zucchini lengthwise in half. Cook, covered in 1 inch boiling salted water 12 to 15 minutes or until tender; drain. Brush with melted Benecol and sprinkle with dill weed.

Easy Baked Beans

Prep Time: 10 Minutes **Baking Time:** 1 Hour
Servings: 6

1 can butter beans, undrained
1 can chili beans
1 can kidney beans, drained
1 chopped onion
¼ cup molasses
¼ cup tomato sauce
1 teaspoon chili powder

Combine all of the above ingredients in a dutch oven and cover. Bake at 325 degrees for 1 hour, removing cover for the last half hour.

Fat Free Fried Rice

Prep Time: 20 Minutes **Cooking Time:** 10 Minutes
Servings: 4

½ cup chicken broth
3 tablespoon sesame seeds
1 cup thinly sliced carrots
1 onion, sliced
2 cloves garlic, minced
1 green pepper, cut into strips
1 cup zucchini, sliced
1 cup mushrooms, sliced
2 cup bean sprouts
1 cup cooked brown rice
1 teaspoon ginger
¼ cup soy sauce
3 tablespoon cilantro, chopped

Heat chicken broth in wok. Add carrots and stir fry for 1 minute over high heat. Mix in onion, garlic, and green pepper; stir fry for 1 more minute. Add zucchini and mushrooms; stir fry until all vegetables are tender-crisp (about 2 more minutes). Mix in bean sprouts and rice and cook until heated through. In a small bowl, mix ginger with soy sauce; blend into rice mixture. Serve immediately, sprinkled with cilantro and sesame seeds.

Fried Rice

Prep Time: 1 Hour **Cooking Time:** 15 Minutes
Servings: 6-8

3 cup brown rice
4 green onions
1 cup chicken
¾ cup egg beaters
Pam Spray
2 cloves garlic, sliced
½ cup soy sauce
1 cup bean sprouts

Cook rice with no salt, let cool. Chop onions, and chicken. Scramble egg beaters in small pan with Pam, add dash of garlic powder. Put eggs aside. In 1 tablespoon of canola oil, fry garlic, remove garlic after it gets brown. Add the rice, stirring constantly, add soy sauce to taste, eggs, and green onions. Add meat and bean sprouts. Serve immediately.

Garlic Broccoli

Prep Time: 10 Minutes **Cooking Time:** 8 Minutes
Servings: 4

3 cup broccoli florets, in bite size pieces
2 teaspoon olive oil
2 cloves garlic
1 red bell pepper, chopped

Steam broccoli and set aside. Heat oil in a medium skillet over medium heat. Add the garlic and bell pepper. Cook, stirring occasionally for 2 minutes. Add the broccoli and cook an additional 2 minutes. Season with salt and pepper and serve.

Green Beans and Almonds

Prep Time: 10 Minutes   **Cooking Time:** 8 Minutes
Servings: 6

1 ½ teaspoon olive oil
1 green onion sliced
½ cup slivered almond
1 ½ pounds green beans
½ teaspoon salt

Heat oil in skillet; add onions and almonds, cook until almonds are golden add the beans and salt. Cook until beans are tender, about 8 minutes.

Grilled Corn on The Cob

Prep Time: 5 Minutes **Chilling:** 1 Hour
Grilling Time: 15 Minutes **Servings:** 6

6 ears of corn with husks
1 gallon ice water

Remove the silks from corn, keeping husks intact. Soak ears in ice water for 1 hour. Remove from water and drain, place on medium heat grill for about 10 minutes turning to grill each side. Remove husks and serve.

Hawaiian Fried Rice

Prep Time: 10 Minutes   **Cooking Time:** 45 Minutes
Servings: 4

3 tablespoon canola oil
½ cup onion, chopped
½ cup raw brown rice
1 tablespoon curry powder
¼ cup raisins
¼ cup chicken broth
¼ cup macadamia nuts, chopped

Heat canola oil in skillet, cook raw rice and onion in pan for a few minutes, stirring well. Add curry, broth and raisins. Cover and bring to boil. Reduce heat, simmer for 40 minutes and add nuts. Stir well, cover and simmer another 5 minutes.

Herb Mushrooms

Prep Time: 15 Minutes **Cooking Time:** 5-10 Minutes
Servings: 4

2 cup fresh mushrooms, halve
¼ cup onion, chopped
2 cloves garlic, minced
2 tablespoon olive oil
1 teaspoon basil
½ teaspoon pepper

In a skillet cook mushrooms, olive oil, onions and garlic over medium heat until mushrooms are tender. Add basil and pepper and heat. Serve.

Herbed Tomatoes
Prep Time: 15 Minutes   Chilling Time: 3 Hours
Servings: 6

6 ripe tomatoes, sliced
1 teaspoon salt
¼ teaspoon freshly ground pepper
½ teaspoon dried thyme or marjoram, crushed
¼ cup finely snipped parsley
¼ cup snipped chives
1/3 cup olive oil
¼ cup tarragon vinegar

Place tomatoes in bowl; sprinkle with seasonings and herbs. Make dressing by combining oil and vinegar; pour over. Cover; chill 3 hours, spooning dressing over a few times. Drain off dressing and pass with tomatoes.

Italian Bean Sauté

Prep Time: 15 Minutes   Servings: 4

4 tablespoon olive oil
2 cloves garlic, minced
1 pound fresh green beans
½ cup chicken broth
5 Roma tomatoes, diced
½ teaspoon basil
½ teaspoon oregano
½ teaspoon rosemary
Salt
Pepper
¼ cup fresh basil, cut loosely
¼ cup fat free grated mozzarella cheese

Heat olive oil in skillet over medium heat. Add garlic and cook for about 1 minute. Add beans continue cooking for 2 minutes, add chicken broth and cook an additional 2 minutes, stir in tomatoes, and seasonings, cook 2-3 minutes monger, just prior to serving add the basil and cheese.

Italian Carrots

Prep Time: 15 Minutes   **Cooking Time:** 10 Minutes
Servings: 6

5 cup carrots sliced
1 tablespoon olive oil
1 green onion, chopped
1 clove garlic, minced
3 tablespoon rice wine vinegar
1½ teaspoon honey
½ teaspoon salt
¼ teaspoon crushed red pepper

Blanch carrots until they are slightly tender, but not fully cooked, about 3-4 minutes. Prepare large skillet by spraying with cooking spray. Heat the oil and add the onions and garlic, cook over medium heat until tender, add the carrots, stir in the remaining ingredients and cook until liquid evaporates.

Lemon Broccoli Pasta

Prep Time: 15 Minutes   **Cooking Time:** 15 Minutes
Serving: 4-6

6 oz of whole wheat spaghetti noodles
2 cup broccoli chopped bite size
2 tablespoon lemon zest
Juice of lemon
¼ cup olive oil
½ cup fat free grated mozzarella cheese
salt and pepper to taste

Prepare noodles as directed on package. In sauce pan cook broccoli until just tender. In a large serving bowl combine the all the ingredients and toss to blend. Serve warm or chilled.

Mozzarella Zucchini

Prep Time: 20 Minutes   **Cooking Time:** 5-10 Minutes
Servings: 4-6

4 c. thinly sliced zucchini
1T water
1 teaspoon salt
1 onion, chopped
2 tablespoon Benecol
Freshly ground pepper
½ cup fat free mozzarella cheese

Put all ingredients except cheese in skillet. Cover and cook 1 minute. Uncover and continue cooking and turning with wide spatula until just tender. About 5 minutes. Sprinkle with cheese. Toss.

Oriental Broccoli

Prep Time: 10 Minutes **Cooking Time:** 10 Minutes
Servings: 4

1 tablespoon fresh ginger root, grated
1 tablespoon soy sauce
1 teaspoon olive oil
1 tablespoon fresh lemon juice
1 tablespoon lemon zest
4 cup broccoli cut into servings
Salt and pepper to taste

Whisk together the ginger, soy sauce, oil, lemon zest, and lemon juice in a shallow serving bowl. Steam broccoli until tender but still crisp. Put broccoli in serving bowl and toss to coat with sauce.

Oven Fried Zucchini

Prep Time: 20 Minutes   **Baking Time:** 10 Minutes
Servings: 4

1 cup whole wheat flour
2 tablespoon cornmeal
1 teaspoon salt
½ teaspoon pepper
3 medium zucchini, sliced lengthwise
2 egg whites, beaten

Prepare a large baking sheet with cooking spray. In a large zip lock bag combine flour, cornmeal, salt and pepper. Dip zucchini in egg whites, shake in the bag to coat and place on pan. Spray the zucchini with cooking spray check to make sure all sides are coated with spray. Bake at 475° for 12 minutes,

Roasted Bell Peppers

Prep Time: 10 Minutes   **Cooking Time:** 15 Minutes
Servings: 4

2 bell peppers
2 teaspoon canola oil

Cut the peppers in half lengthwise. And brush with oil. Broil in oven until skins are charred. Cover tightly for 10 minutes. Remove skins with your fingers and a knife and serve.

Red Beans and Rice

Prep Time: 20 Minutes **Baking Time:** 30 Minutes
Servings: 6

2 cup brown rice, cooked
1 can kidney beans
1 cup salsa
2 tablespoon green onions, chopped
2 tablespoon jalapeno peppers, minced (optional)

Preheat oven to 350 degrees. Mix rice, beans and salsa add jalapenos if desired, in a casserole dish. Top with green onions. Bake for 30 Minutes.

Rice Pilaf

Prep Time: 30 Minutes **Baking Time:** 1 Hour
Servings: 4

1 (4 oz.) can mushrooms
2 teaspoon oregano flakes
¼ cup Benecol
2 cup brown rice, uncooked
8 green onions, sliced
3 cans beef broth
2 cans water
Salt & pepper to taste

Sauté onions and rice in Benecol until rice is lightly brown. Add oregano and mushrooms. Put in large casserole and add liquid. Bake in hot oven at 450 degrees for about 45 minutes to 1 hour or until liquid is absorbed. Cover casserole.

Roasted Sweet Potatoes

Prep Time: 15 Minutes   **Baking Time:** 1 Hour
Servings: 6

3 sweet potatoes, cut in 1½ inch pieces.
2 tablespoon olive oil
Onion powder
Garlic salt
Pepper

Prepare baking pan by lightly spraying with cooking spray. Place potatoes in pan in a single layer, brush with olive oil and sprinkle with spices. Bake cover at 325° for 45 minutes and uncovered for another 15 minutes.

Sautéed Spinach

Prep Time: 2 Minutes   **Cooking Time:** 10 Minutes
Servings: 4

2 tablespoon olive oil
8 cup fresh spinach
2 tablespoon balsamic vinegar
Salt and pepper to taste

In large skillet heat oil over medium heat add spinach, cook until wilted add vinegar and salt and pepper.

Sautéed Spinach and Mushroom
Prep Time: 10 Minutes   Cooking Time: 10 Minutes
Servings: 4

8 cup fresh spinach, washed
1½ cup Mushrooms sliced
2 tablespoon olive oil
2 cloves garlic minced
Salt and pepper to taste
In large skillet heat oil and garlic, add mushroom and spinach, cook over medium heat for about 10 minutes or until the mushrooms are tender, add salt and pepper to taste.

Sautéed Squash

Prep Time: 10 Minutes **Cooking Time:** 10 Minutes
Servings: 4

2 teaspoon olive oil
4 green onions, sliced thin
½ green bell pepper, sliced
1 yellow squash sliced
1 zucchini, sliced
¼ teaspoon cayenne pepper
½ teaspoon salt
½ teaspoon pepper

Heat oil in a medium skillet over medium heat; add the green onions and bell pepper, cooking for 3 minutes stirring often. Add the squash and zucchini and cook until softened. Add the remaining spices and toss.

Savory Baked Beans

Prep Time: 15 Minutes **Cooking/Baking Time:** 2 hours and 45 minutes **Servings:** 4

1 cup dry navy, marrow or other beans
3 cup water
1 bay leaf
1 clove garlic, minced
1 onion, chopped
1 T. chopped parsley
½ cup finely diced celery
1 tablespoon canola oil
1 can (8 1/4 oz.) stewed tomatoes, mashed
½ teaspoon dried basil leaves, crumbled
½ teaspoon salt
1/8 teaspoon black pepper

Wash beans. Put in large saucepan with the water. Bring to a boil. Boil for 2 minutes. Cover. Let stand for 1 hour. Add bay leaf, garlic, onion and parsley, bring to boil again. Cover loosely. Simmer for 45 minutes or until beans are just tender. Put beans in 1½ quart casserole. Meanwhile, sauté celery in oil for about 5 minutes. Add tomatoes, basil, salt and pepper. Bring to a boil. Simmer 10 minutes, stirring occasionally. Stir mixture into beans. Cover. Bake at 250 degrees for 2 hours.

Savory Asparagus

Prep Time: 10 Minutes **Baking Time:** 10 minutes
Servings: 4

1 pound asparagus
Olive oil
Garlic salt
Onion powder
Salt
Pepper

Prepare baking sheet by lightly spraying with cooking spray. Lay asparagus out on cooking sheet in one layer. Brush with olive oil and sprinkle with spices. Bake at 350° for 10 minutes or until vegetables are tender.

Spanish Rice

Prep Time: 10 Minutes   **Cooking Time:** 50 Minutes
Servings: 6

1 can beef broth and 1 can water
½ cup green onion, chopped
1 tomato, chopped
½ teaspoon salt
¼ teaspoon pepper
¼ teaspoon garlic powder
¼ teaspoon cumin
1 cup brown rice
1 tablespoon canola oil

Brown rice in oil, add broth and water to rice; cover and cook until liquid is absorbed, about 50 minutes. Add the rest of the ingredients. Mix and serve.

Spicy Black Beans

Prep Time: 1 Hour **Soaking and Cooking Time:** 4 Hours **Servings:** 4-6

½ pound black beans
1 onion, chopped
1 teaspoon salt
1/8 teaspoon oregano
4 tablespoon olive oil
1 green pepper, chopped
2 cloves garlic, minced
Dash of pepper
1 teaspoon honey
1 bay leaf
1 teaspoon vinegar

Wash beans. Soak 3 hours in 2 quarts of water. Bring beans to a boil in same water and simmer on low heat for 1 hour. Heat oil and add garlic, green pepper and onion. Add oregano, bay leaf, salt, honey and pepper. Cook 10 minutes. Add to beans when they are well cooked. Add vinegar. Serve with cooked brown rice.

Spicy Rice

Prep Time: 15 Minutes **Cooking Time:** 15 Minutes
Servings: 4

½ cup green onions, sliced
½ cup carrots, minced
½ cup red pepper. minced
1 jalapeno and serrano pepper, minced
1 tablespoon canola oil
2 cup cooked brown rice (cooked in chicken broth)
2 tablespoon snipped cilantro
1 tablespoon lime juice
1 teaspoon soy sauce
Tabasco sauce to taste

Cook onions, carrots, red pepper and jalapeno pepper in oil in large skillet over medium high heat until tender crisp. Stir in rice, cilantro, lime juice, soy sauce, and Tabasco cook until thoroughly heated.

Spicy Tomato Juice

Prep Time: 15 Minutes **Chilling Time:** 2 Hours
Servings: 2 Servings

2 cup tomato juice
1 teaspoon grated onion
½ teaspoon celery salt
1 tablespoon lemon juice
1 teaspoon Worcestershire sauce
½ teaspoon salt
½ teaspoon paprika
Dash garlic slat

Mix together all ingredients, let chill for 2 hours and serve.

Spicy Zucchini

Prep Time: 15 Minutes **Baking Time:** 30 Minutes
Servings: 4

2 cloves garlic
2 tablespoon olive oil
½ teaspoon rosemary
½ teaspoon thyme
½ teaspoon pepper
¼ teaspoon red pepper flakes
½ salt
2-3 small zucchini, sliced

In a saucepan heat oil and garlic, cook for 2 minutes add other spices. Drizzle over zucchini and toss to coat. Place zucchini in a baking pan. Bake at 350° for 30 minutes or until zucchini is tender.

Sautéed Vegetables

Prep Time: 10 Minutes **Cooking Time:** 10 Minutes
Servings: 4

2 green peppers, seeded and cut into strips
2 onions, sliced
2 cup fresh mushrooms, sliced
2 tablespoon canola oil
Salt and pepper

Heat oil in large skillet and sauté until vegetables are tender, salt and pepper.

Sweet Pepper Relish

Prep Time: 10 Minutes   Cooking Time: 7 Minutes
Servings: 4-6

1/3 cup apple cider vinegar
2 tablespoon honey
½ teaspoon dry mustard
½ teaspoon salt
½ teaspoon allspice
1 green bell pepper, chopped
1 red bell pepper chopped
½ cup onion, chopped

Combine all the ingredients in a small sauce pan, bring to boil over medium heat. Reduce heat and cook for about for another 10 minutes. Serve with chicken or fish.

Sweet Rice

**Prep Time: 20 Minutes   Cooking Time: 15 Minutes
Servings: 6-8**

½ cup chopped celery
½ cup chopped onions
1 tablespoon Benecol
1/8 teaspoon allspice
1/8 teaspoon cinnamon
1/8 teaspoon salt
1 tablespoon molasses
3 cup cooked brown rice
½ cup raisins plumped
1 tart apple, cored and chopped
½ cup sliced almonds

In a large skillet cook celery and onions in Benecol until tender. Stir in seasonings, rice and raisins. Heat thoroughly. Stir in apple, cored and chopped. Remove from heat. Cover and let stand 5 minutes. Sprinkle with almonds.

Tasty Brown Rice

Prep Time: 15 Minutes   **Cooking Time:** 60 Minutes
Servings: 6-8

3 cup brown rice
6 cup water
¼ cup olive oil
Salt
2 onions, chopped
6 chicken bouillon cubes
4 cloves garlic, minced

Put all ingredients in 3-quart saucepan. Cover. Bring to a boil stir once, turn heat to low and simmer for 50 minutes. Remove rice from heat and allow to sit for 10 minutes, serve.

Vegetable Rice

Prep Time: 20 Minutes   **Cooking Time:** 15 Minutes
Servings: 6-8

1 cup onion, chopped
2 zucchinis, sliced
3 tablespoon olive oil
1 can diced tomatoes
1 can corn, drained
3 cup cooked brown rice
1½ teaspoon salt
¼ teaspoon pepper
¼ teaspoon ground coriander
¼ teaspoon oregano

In a sauce pan sauté onions and zucchini in olive oil. Add other ingredients. Cover and simmer 15 minutes.

Vegetable Stir Fry
Prep Time: 30 Minutes **Cooking Time:** 10 Minutes
Servings: 6

¼ cup cold water
1 tablespoon corn starch
2 tablespoon soy sauce
½ tablespoon honey
1 tablespoon lemon juice
½ teaspoon salt
¼ teaspoon pepper
1½ tablespoon canola oil
2 teaspoon fresh ginger grated
1 cup fresh green beans
1 ½ cup cauliflower
1 ½ cup broccoli
1 onion chopped coarsely
½ cup slice carrots
1 small zucchini, sliced
1 cup bean sprouts

Combine water and corn starch, stir in soy sauce, lemon juice, honey, and salt and pepper, set aside. Pour oil into wok and heat over medium high heat, add ginger to flavor oil. Add onion, carrots, allow to cook for 2 minutes. Add beans cauliflower and broccoli, cook an additional 2 minutes. Add zucchini and bean sprouts, cook 1 minute, add sauce to center of wok. Cook and stir until thickened. Serve.

Vegetable Fried Rice

Prep Time: 30 Minutes   **Cooking Time:** 60 Minutes
Servings: 4

1 cup brown rice
1 bag frozen vegetables (broccoli, carrots & cauliflower mix)
1 tablespoon seasoned salt
Garlic powder
2 tablespoon canola oil
½ cup egg beaters
¼ teaspoon black pepper
¼ c soy sauce

Cook rice as directed on package. Heat oil in frying pan; add frozen vegetables and stir fry until lightly tender. Beat egg beaters and add to vegetables (scrambling time). Add cooked rice and seasonings. Stir fry until golden brown. Add soy sauce.

Vegetable Wrap
Prep Time: 15 Minutes   Servings: 6

2 avocados, peeled and chopped
2 large tomatoes, chopped
½ cup red onion, minced
2 tablespoon jalapeno, minced
2 tablespoon fresh cilantro, chopped
2 tablespoon olive oil
2 tablespoon lemon juice
2 tablespoon lime juice
1 teaspoon cumin
1 teaspoon chili powder
1 can black beans, drained
1 cup lettuce, shredded
6 whole wheat tortilla shells
Salt and pepper to taste

Put the avocados, tomatoes, onion, jalapeno, beans and cilantro in a mixing bowl, toss to mix, and set aside. In a small bowl, whisk the olive oil, juices, cumin, chili powder, salt and pepper. Add to the avocado mixture and toss gently. Spoon avocado mixture into heated tortilla and add lettuce. Roll and serve.

Vietnamese Fried Rice

Prep Time: 30 Minutes   **Cooking Time:** 8 Minutes
Servings: 4-6

2 tablespoon peanut oil
1 onion, chopped
½ cup egg beaters, made into an omelet and chopped finely
½ cup green onions, chopped
5 cup cooked brown rice, chill overnight
3 tablespoon soy sauce
1 tablespoon honey
1 cup fresh bean sprouts

Heat up a wok or heavy fry pan with oil until hot. Add onion and stir fry for 1 minute. Add egg beaters, scallions and rice, stir until mixed well. Add soy sauce, and honey stir for 5 to 8 minutes. Add bean sprouts, and stir for 2 more minutes.

Western Baked Beans

Prep Time: 30 Minutes **Baking Time:** 30 Minutes
Servings: 6

½ pound ground buffalo
1 cup onion, chopped
2 teaspoon salt, dash pepper
½ cup tomato paste
1 tablespoon vinegar
1 tablespoon mustard
2 cans beans (in tomato sauce)

Using a skillet, brown buffalo and onions. Add remaining ingredients. Pour into baking dish. Bake at 400 degrees for 30 minutes.

Chapter 16
Desserts

Apple Brownies
Apple Cake
Apple Oatmeal Cookies
Applesauce Loaf
Applesauce Oatmeal Cookies
Baked Apples
Baked Orange Apples
Banana Oatmeal Crispies
Blackberry Crisps
Blueberry Streusel Muffins
Brownies
Brownies
Carrot Cake
Cherry Cobbler
Chocolate Chip Cookies
Chocolate Chip Cookie Strips
Chocolate Covered Strawberries
Chocolate Krinkle Cookies
Chocolate Nut Fondue
Chocolate Puffs

Fantastic Peanut Butter Cookies
Fresh Fruit Pizza
Frozen Chocolate Bananas
Fudge Squares
Gingersnaps
Grilled Apples
Hermits
Honey Lemon Cookies
Lemon Streusel
Nut Chocolate Cookies
Oatmeal Chocolate Chip Cookies
Oatmeal Cookies
Oatmeal Molasses Cockies
Peach Berry Supreme
Pecan Delights
Rice Pudding
Spice Cake
Stuffed Pears
Sweet Potato Soufflé

Apple Brownies

Prep Time: 20 Minutes   **Baking Time:** 40 Minutes
Servings: 9

1/4 cup coconut oil
1 cup whole wheat flour
1 cup evaporated cane juice
1 egg white
1 teaspoon baking soda
1 cup apples, chopped & peeled
1 cup chopped walnuts
1 teaspoon cinnamon

Preheat oven to 350°. Melt coconut oil in a pan. Combine other ingredients and mix with coconut oil. Pour into sprayed with cooking spray 8 x 8 inch dish. Bake for approximately 40 minutes. Cool and cut into squares.

Apple Cake

Prep Time: 25 Minutes   **Baking Time:** 30 Minutes
Servings: 6-8

2 egg whites
½ cup molasses
½ cup honey
1 teaspoon vanilla
¼ teaspoon salt
½ cup whole wheat pastry flour,
2 teaspoon baking powder
2 apples, pared then chopped or sliced
½ cup walnuts or pecans, chopped

Beat egg whites in a medium size bowl; then add honey and molasses, vanilla, salt, flour, apples and nuts. Spread it all in a greased 9 inch pie plate and bake for 30 minutes at 350°.

Apple Oatmeal Cookies
Prep Time: 20 Minutes   Baking Time: 12 Minutes
Servings: 2½ Dozen

¾ cup honey
½ cup coconut oil
2 cup oats
2 teaspoon cinnamon
½ teaspoon salt
½ cup nuts, chopped
3 egg whites
1 teaspoon vanilla
1 cup whole wheat flour
½ teaspoon baking soda
1 teaspoon baking powder
1 apple, shredded

Heat oven to 375°. Beat together honey and coconut oil. Beat in egg whites and vanilla. Add combined dry ingredients, mix well. Stir in apple and nuts. Drop on cookie sheet, sprayed with cooking spray. Bake 9 to 12 minutes. Cool 1 minute on cookie sheet; remove to wire cooling rack. Store in tightly covered container.

Applesauce Loaf

Prep Time: 25 Minutes **Baking Time:** 60 Minutes
Servings: 8

2 cup whole wheat pastry flour
1 teaspoon baking soda
1 teaspoon cinnamon
1 teaspoon baking powder
1 cup applesauce
¾ cup honey
3 egg whites
½ cup Smart Balance, melted
½ cup raisins

Heat oven to 350°. In a medium bowl combine flour, baking soda, cinnamon and baking powder. In a large bowl blend applesauce, honey, egg whites and Smart Balance. Stir in flour mixture just until blended. Batter will be lumpy. Mix in raisins. Spoon batter into sprayed loaf pan. Bake 55 to 60 minutes or until toothpick inserted in center comes out clean. Cool.

Applesauce Oatmeal Cookies
Prep Time: 15 Minutes   **Baking Time:** 8 Minutes
Servings: 28

1/3 cup coconut oil
½ cup honey
1 teaspoon cinnamon
¼ teaspoon baking soda
1 egg white
½ cup unsweetened applesauce
1¼ cup whole wheat flour
1¼ cup rolled oats

In large mixing bowl combine coconut oil, honey, cinnamon and soda. Beat until combined. Add eggs and applesauce, beat. Add flour mix, stir in oats. Drop by dough by rounded teaspoons about 2 inches apart on ungreased cookie sheet. Bake at 375° for 8-10 minutes.

Baked Apples

Prep Time: 15 Minutes   **Baking Time:** 40 Minutes
Servings: 4

4 medium apples (tart apples like Jonathan or Granny Smith)
½ cup raisins
½ cup pecans (chopped)
2 tablespoon honey
1 teaspoon cinnamon
½ teaspoon nutmeg
1/3 cup water

Core apples and place them in a casserole dish. Combine raisins, nuts, honey, cinnamon and nutmeg. Spoon into center of apples. Pour water into casserole. Bake at 350° for 40-45 minutes or until apples are tender. Serve warm.

Baked Orange Apples

Prep Time: 15 Minutes   **Baking Time:** 30 Minutes
Servings: 4

4 baking apples
1 cup water
1 orange, sliced
¼ cup unsweetened apple juice
1 teaspoon cinnamon
1 tablespoon honey

Preheat oven to 350°. Core the apples and remove one-fourth of the top peel. Place apples in a shallow baking pan. Combine the water, juice honey and cinnamon. Pour over the apples. Arrange the orange slices around the apples to help flavor the liquid. Cover the pan with aluminum foil and bake about 20 to 30 minutes or until fork tender.

Banana Oatmeal Crispies

Prep Time: 25 Minutes **Baking Time:** 20-25 Minutes
Servings: 2½ Dozen

2 cup quick oats
½ cup unsweetened coconut
¾ cup chopped dated
2 teaspoon soy flour
¼ cup whole wheat flour
1 ripe mashed banana
1/3 cup canola oil
½ teaspoon salt
1 tablespoon vanilla
¼ cup water

Mix the first six ingredients together. Whiz remaining ingredients in blender. Add whizzed mixture to dry ingredients and mix well. Let stand 10 minutes. Spoon onto greased cookie sheet. Bake at 375° for 20-25 minutes or until nicely browned.

Blackberry Crisps

Prep Time: 15 Minutes **Baking Time:** 45 Minutes
Servings: 8

1 cup oats, quick cooking
¾ cup whole wheat pastry flour
2 teaspoon cinnamon
½ cup benecol, melted
3 cup frozen blackberries, thawed
1 tablespoon orange juice
¼ cup honey

Mix the oats, 1/2 cup of the flour, 1 teaspoon cinnamon and melted benecol until crumbly in texture. Spray an 8 x 8 inch baking pan and place half of the mixture in the bottom. Retain second half for topping. Combine the blackberries, orange juice, honey and remaining ¼ cup flour and remaining teaspoon of cinnamon. Spread over the oat mixture. Cover with remaining half of the oat mixture. Bake at 350° for 45 minutes.

Blueberry Streusel Muffins

Prep Time: 20 Minutes **Baking Time:** 18-20 Minutes
Servings: 8

2 cup flour
¾ cup flour
2½ teaspoon baking powder
¾ teaspoon salt
¼ Benecol
¾ cup skim milk
1 egg white
2 cup blueberries
Topping
½ cup stevia
1/3 cup flour
½ teaspoon cinnamon
¼ cup Benecol

Mix all ingredients, spoon into muffin pan with muffin liners. Sprinkle with topping. Bake at 350° 18 to 20 minutes.

Brownies

Prep Time: 20 Minutes   **Baking Time:** 25 Minutes
Servings: 8

½ cup honey
1/3 cup water
3 tablespoon canola oil
½ teaspoon vanilla extract
2 egg whites, lightly beaten
½ cup whole wheat flour
1/3 cup quick cooking oats, uncooked
¼ cup unsweetened cocoa
2 teaspoon baking powder
1/8 teaspoon salt

Combine honey, water, oil, and vanilla in a medium bowl; stir well. Add egg whites, and stir well. Combine flour and next 4 ingredients; add to honey mixture, stirring well. Pour batter into an 8 inch square baking pan coated with cooking spray. Bake at 350° for 23 minutes or until wooden pick inserted in center comes out clean. Cool.

Brownies

Prep Time: 20 Minutes **Baking Time:** 25 Minutes
Servings: 8-12

1/2 cup coconut oil
½ cup Xocia Juice
1 cup evaporated cane juice
2 egg whites
½ cup whole wheat flour
½ teaspoon baking powder
½ teaspoon salt
½ cup chopped pecans

Combine coconut oil and chocolate. Beat in cane juice and slightly beaten egg whites. Combine the flour, baking powder and salt together and add to creamed mixture. Add vanilla and beat well. Add nuts. Put mixture in pan sprayed with Pan. Bake at 325 degrees for 25 to 30 minutes. Brownies are done when they pull away from edge of pan.

Carrot Cake

**Prep Time: 30 Minutes   Baking Time: 35-45 Minutes
Servings: 12-15**

2 cup whole wheat flour
2 teaspoon baking powder
1 teaspoon soda
1 teaspoon cinnamon
1 cup honey
3 cup shredded carrots
½ cup canola oil
½ cup fat free yogurt
3 egg whites

Spray and lightly flour 9 X 13 inch baking pan. In large mixing bowl combine dry ingredients. Add carrots, honey, oil, and egg beaters. Beat until combined. Pour batter into the pan. Bake at 350° for 35-40 minutes or until a toothpick comes out clean.

Cherry Cobbler

Prep Time: 25 Minutes   **Baking Time:** 35-40 Minutes
Servings: 8

6 tablespoon Benecol
1 cup whole wheat pastry flour
1½ teaspoon baking powder
1½ cup honey
½ cup skim milk
1½ cup boiling water
2 cup cherries

Melt 4 tablespoon Benecol in baking dish. Combine flour, baking powder 2 tablespoon Benecol, ½ cup honey and the milk to make dough. Pour dough over melted Benecol. Add boiling water. Add remaining honey and cherries. Bake at 400° for 35-40 minutes.

Chocolate Chip Cookies

Prep Time: 15 Minutes **Baking Time:** 10 Minutes
Servings: 2 Dozen

½ cup coconut oil
¾ cup evaporated cane juice
1 teaspoon vanilla
2 egg whites
1½ cup whole wheat flour
½ teaspoon baking soda
1 teaspoon baking powder
1 teaspoon salt
1 cup dark chocolate chips
½ cup unsweetened coconut
½ cup chopped walnuts

Cream coconut oil and evaporated cane juice; add egg whites. Combine flour, soda and salt together; Add to creamed mixture; add vanilla, chocolate chips, coconut and walnuts. Drop by teaspoonfuls; bake 10 to 15 minutes at 350°.

Chocolate Chip Cookie Strips

Prep Time: 30 Minutes **Baking Time:** 9 Minutes
Servings: 2½ Dozen

¾ cup evaporated cane juice
½ cup canola oil
1 teaspoon vanilla
2 egg whites
1½ cup whole wheat flour
½ teaspoon soda
1 teaspoon baking powder
1 teaspoon salt
1 cup dark chocolate chips
½ cup chopped nuts

Mix evaporated cane juice, oil, vanilla and egg whites. Stir until smooth. Stir in flour and other dry ingredients. Divide dough into 2 strips, about 15 x 2 inches. Place about 3 inches apart on cookie sheet, sprayed with cooking spray. Sprinkle each strip with chocolate chips and nuts. Press lightly. Bake until golden brown at 375° for 7 to 9 minutes. Cool 2 minutes. Cut each strip crosswise into 1 inch slices; repeat with remaining dough.

Chocolate Covered Strawberries
Prep Time: 15 Minutes Cooking Time: 10 Minutes
Servings: 12

1 dark chocolate bar
½ teaspoon vanilla
12 Strawberries with stems

Melt chocolate in top of double boiler. Blend in vanilla. Dip strawberries in chocolate, swirling to coat evenly. Place on waxed paper and set in cool dry place.

Chocolate Krinkle Cookies

Prep Time: 15 Minutes   **Baking Time:** 15 Minutes
Servings: 12

½ cup cocoa
¾ cup evaporated cane juice
3 tablespoon coconut oil
1½ teaspoon vanilla
1 egg white
1 tablespoon skim milk
½ cup whole wheat flour
½ teaspoon salt
1 teaspoon baking powder
½ cup walnuts, chopped

Heat oven to 350°. Mix evaporated cane juice, coconut oil, vanilla and egg whites in medium bowl. Stir in cocoa and milk. Stir in flour, salt, and baking powder. Stir in walnuts. Drop dough by tablespoonfuls about 3 inches apart onto lightly sprayed cookie sheet. Bake 13 to 15 minutes. Cool slightly before removing from cookie sheet.

Chocolate Nut Fondue

Prep Time: 10 Minutes   **Cooking Time:** 10 Minutes
Servings: 4-6

1 dark chocolate bar
½ cup honey
½ cup skim milk
½ cup chunky peanut butter

In saucepan combine chocolate, honey and milk. Cook, stirring constantly until heated through. Add peanut butter; mix well. Pour into fondue pot; place over fondue burner. Spear dipper with fork, dip in sauce. Suggested dippers: bananas, apples, cherries, pineapple, strawberries.

Chocolate Puffs

Prep Time: 30 Minutes   **Baking Time:** 10 Minutes
Servings: 3 Dozen

½ cup cocoa
2 egg whites
½ teaspoon salt
½ cup evaporated can juice
½ teaspoon vanilla
½ teaspoon vinegar
¾ cup chopped walnuts

Beat egg whites with salt until foamy. Gradually add evaporated cane juice; beat until stiff peaks form. Beat in vanilla and vinegar. Fold in cocoa and walnuts. Drop by teaspoonful onto cookie sheet sprayed with cooking spray. Bake 350° for 10 minutes. Remove immediately.

Fantastic Peanut Butter Cookies

Prep Time: 10 Minutes **Baking Time:** 8 Minutes
Servings: 2 Dozen

2 egg whites, beaten
1 cup evaporated cane juice
1 cup peanut butter

Mix beaten egg whites and evaporated cane juice together, then add peanut butter. Roll into a ball about size of a walnut crisscross with fork. Bake at 350° for 8 minutes They burn very easy, watch closely.

Fresh Fruit Pizza

Prep Time: 35 Minutes **Baking Time:** 18 Minutes
Servings: 6-8

Crust
½ cup coconut oil
½ cup honey
3 egg whites
1 teaspoon vanilla
1¼ cup whole wheat pastry flour
½ cup oat flour
2 teaspoon baking powder
1 teaspoon soda
1 teaspoon salt
1 cup pecans, chopped
¼ cup unsweetened coconut
Filling
1 8 oz package fat free cream cheese
2 tablespoon honey
1 cup strawberries
Toppings
1 apple
2 bananas
2 kiwis
6 fresh strawberries
1 cup pineapple chunks

Cream oil and honey until light. Beat in eggs and vanilla. Combine dry ingredients; blend into creamed mixture. Stir in nuts and coconut. Spread on pizza pan or cookie sheet with sides, sprayed with Pam. Bake at 375° for 18 minutes. Cool slightly. In food processor blend all filling ingredients until smooth, spread on crust and top with fruit.

Frozen Chocolate Bananas

Prep Time: 15 Minutes   **Freezing Time:** 3 Hours
Servings: 8

Chopped peanuts
1 dark chocolate bar
4 Bananas

Place peanuts in a bowl. Put a piece of waxed paper on a plate. 2. Melt chocolate, stir until melted. Remove from heat. Peel banana. Cut banana in half. Push a wooden stick into end of each banana half (popsicle sticks will work). Dip or spread Nugget sauce on all sides of banana halves. Roll in peanuts to coat. Put bananas on waxed paper. Freeze until hard. If you want to save for another day, wrap in plastic wrap.

Fudge Squares

Prep Time: 20 Minutes   **Baking Time:** 35 Minutes
Servings: 12-15

1 cup whole wheat flour
2 teaspoon baking powder
1 teaspoon salt
2/3 cup coconut oil
½ cup cocoa
1 cup evaporated cane juice
4 egg whites
½ cup skim milk
2 teaspoon vanilla
1 cup walnuts

Combine baking powder, salt and flour. Put coconut oil and cocoa in mixing bowl and mix well; add evaporated cane juice gradually add egg whites while beating. Fold in flour mixture. Add milk, vanilla and nuts and mix well. Bake in 9 x 13 inch pan sprayed with Pam at 325° for 35 minutes.

Gingersnaps

Prep Time: 25 Minutes   **Baking Time:** 8 minutes
Servings: 36

2¼ cup whole wheat flour
½ cup honey
½ cup coconut oil
¼ cup nonfat plain yogurt
¼ cup molasses
1 egg white
1 teaspoon baking soda
1 teaspoon ginger
1 teaspoon cinnamon
½ teaspoon cloves

In large mixing bowl combine half the flour, oil, yogurt, honey, molasses, egg, baking soda, ginger, cinnamon, and cloves. Beat on medium speed until combined. Beat in additional flour. Shape dough in 1 inch balls. Place balls 2 inches apart on ungreased cookie sheet. Bake at 375° for 8-10 minutes. Cool cookies on sheet for 1 minute before transferring them to a cooling rack.

Grilled Apples

**Prep Time: 20 Minutes   Cooking Time: 30 Minutes
Servings: 4**

4 Baking apples
2 tablespoon Benecol
2 tablespoon honey
1 teaspoon cinnamon
1 teaspoon Freshly grated nutmeg
½ cup chopped walnuts

Use one square of heavy duty foil for each apple, make it large enough to wrap an apple. Core apples. Place an apple on each square of foil and fill core cavity with a ½ tablespoon Benecol, a ½ tablespoon honey, sprinkle of cinnamon and a pinch of nutmeg and a few chopped nuts. Pull up foil around apple and bake until done over hot grill about 30 minutes.

Hermits

Prep Time: 25 Minutes   **Baking Time:** 10 Minutes
Servings: 36

½ cup coconut oil
½ cup honey
½ teaspoon baking soda
½ teaspoon cinnamon
¼ teaspoon nutmeg
¼ teaspoon ground cloves
1 egg white
2 tablespoon skim milk
1 teaspoon vanilla
1½ cup whole wheat flour
1 cup raisins
½ cup chopped nuts

Spray cookie sheet, set aside. In mixing bowl better oil, honey, baking soda, cinnamon, nutmeg and cloves. Beat until combined. Scraping sides occasionally. Add eggs, milk, and vanilla, beat until combined. Add flour and mix, stir in raisins and nuts. Drop by rounded teaspoons about 2 inches apart on cookie sheet. Press down with fingers. Bake at 375° for 10 minutes. Cool on wire rack.

Honey Lemon Cookies

Prep Time: 20 Minutes **Set Time:** overnight
Baking Time: 8-10 Minutes **Servings:** 24

2¼ cup whole wheat flour
1 teaspoon soda
1 teaspoon baking powder
½ cup honey
½ cup molasses
3 egg whites
1 teaspoon vanilla
1 teaspoon lemon extract

Mix and let stand overnight at room temperature. In the morning, roll out and cut with doughnut cutter and bake at 350° for 8-10 minutes.

Lemon Streusel

Prep Time: 30 Minutes **Baking Time:** 35-40 Minutes
Servings: 8

2¼ cup whole wheat pastry flour
3 teaspoon baking powder
½ teaspoon salt
¾ cup honey
1 cup nonfat plain yogurt
3 tablespoon canola oil
1 tablespoon fresh lemon juice
1 tablespoon grated lemon peel
½ teaspoon vanilla
4 egg whites, stiffly beaten
Streusel
¼ cup evaporated cane juice granules
¼ cup uncooked oats

Mix flour, baking powder and salt. Beat honey, yogurt, oil, lemon juice, grated lemon peel and vanilla. Add dry ingredients. Fold in beaten egg whites. Pour into cupcake papers. Top with streusel. Bake at 350° for 35 to 40 minutes.

Nut Chocolate Cookies

Prep Time: 30 Minutes **Cooking Time:** 10 Minutes
Servings: 48 cookies

½ cup coconut oil
1 cup evaporated cane juice
2 egg whites, lightly beaten
1 tablespoon skim milk
1 t. vanilla extract
1 C. whole wheat pastry flour
1 t. baking powder
½ teaspoon baking soda
½ teaspoon salt
1 cup quick-cooking oats
½ cup cocoa
1 c. coarsely chopped walnuts

Cream the coconut oil and evaporated cane juice in a large mixer bowl until light and fluffy. Add egg whites, milk and vanilla and beat until blended. Combine the flour, baking powder, baking soda and salt together and add to the creamed mixture. Stir just until blended. Stir in the oats. Fold in the cocoa and walnuts. Refrigerate the dough covered for at least 1 hour. Preheat oven to 350 degrees. Spray cookie sheet with Pam. Shape the dough into balls, using a teaspoon for small cookies or a tablespoon for large cookies. Flatten slightly, place 2 inches apart on the prepared baking sheets. Bake until the edges are slightly browned, about 10 minutes. Don't overbake, because the cookies do harden as they cool. Remove from the oven and let cool on the sheets for 10 minutes. Remove to wire racks to cool completely.

Oatmeal Chocolate Chip Cookies
Prep Time: 30 Minutes **Baking Time:** 8 Minutes
Servings: 6 Dozen

1½ cup whole wheat pastry flour
1 teaspoon baking powder
1 teaspoon soda
1 teaspoon salt
¾ cup coconut oil
1 cup evaporated cane juice
3 egg whites
1 cup nuts
1½ cup dark chocolate chips
2 cup oatmeal
2 teaspoon vanilla

Cream coconut oil and cane juice; add egg whites and blend well. Combine flour, soda and salt together; add to creamed ingredients. Mix nuts, chocolate chips and oatmeal together and add to mixture; add vanilla. Drop by teaspoonfuls; bake 8 to 10 minutes at 375 degrees.

Oatmeal Cookies

Prep Time: 25 Minutes   **Baking Time:** 10 Minutes
Servings: 36

½ cup coconut oil
¼ cup fat free yogurt
¾ cup honey
2 teaspoon baking powder
¼ teaspoon baking soda
1 teaspoon cinnamon
¼ teaspoon ground cloves
2 egg whites
1 teaspoon vanilla
1¾ cup whole wheat flour
2 cup rolled oats
1 cup chopped nuts
1 cup raisins (optional)

In large mixing bowl combine coconut oil, honey, baking powder, soda, and spices. Beat until combined. Add egg whites and vanilla, beat. Add flour mix, add oats, nuts and raisins, stir. Drop by dough by rounded teaspoons about 2 inches apart on ungreased cookie sheet. Bake at 375° for 10-12 minutes.

Oatmeal Molasses Cookies
Prep Time: 20 Minutes   Baking Time: 10 Minutes
Servings: 2 Dozen

1 ½ cup whole wheat flour
1 teaspoon soda
1 teaspoon baking powder
1 teaspoon salt
½ teaspoon cloves
½ teaspoon ginger
1 cup evaporated cane juice
¾ cup coconut oil
2 egg whites
¼ cup molasses
¾ cup quick oatmeal

Cream evaporated cane juice and coconut oil. Add egg whites and beat. Add molasses. Then add combined dry ingredients. Stir in oatmeal. Drop by teaspoonfuls 2 inches apart. Bake at 375° for 8 to 10 minutes.

Peach Cobbler

Prep Time: 15 Minutes   **Baking Time:** 45 Minutes
Servings: 8

1 cup whole wheat pastry flour
1 teaspoon baking powder
½ teaspoon salt
½ cup evaporated cane juice
1 cup skim milk
2 teaspoon Benecol
1 can peaches (canned in fruit juice, no added sugar)

Melt Benecol in 8X8 baking pan. Blend flour, baking powder, salt, honey and milk and pour over Benecol. Then pour in large can of peaches. Cook at 400° for 45 minutes to an hour.

Peach Berry Supreme
Prep Time: 15 Minutes **Baking Time:** 30 Minutes
Servings: 6

3 cup fresh raspberries
2 cup sliced peaches
¼ cup honey
1 tablespoon whole wheat flour
¼ teaspoon ginger
5 cup soft whole wheat bread crumbs
3 tablespoon Benecol

Combine flour and ginger in a mixing bowl, add the honey and fruit, toss to coat. Add 2 cup of the bread crumbs, toss gently to combine. Put fruit mixture in a baking dish. Place remaining bread crumbs in a mixing bowl, drizzle with melted Benecol, toss to coat. Sprinkle bread crumbs over fruit mixture. Bake at 375° for 30 minutes.

Pecan Delights

Prep Time: 30 minutes **Baking Time:** 10 Minutes
Servings: 2½ dozen

½ cup coconut oil
½ cup honey
3 egg whites
1 teaspoon vanilla
1¼ cup whole wheat pastry flour
½ cup oat flour
2 teaspoon baking powder
1 teaspoon soda
1 teaspoon salt
1 cup pecans, chopped

Cream oil and honey until light. Beat in eggs and vanilla. Combine dry ingredients; blend into creamed mixture. Stir in nuts and coconut. Drop from teaspoon on ungreased cookie sheet. Bake at 375° about 10 minutes. Cool cookies slightly before removing from cookie sheet.

Rice Pudding

Prep Time: 20 Minutes   **Cooking Time:** 45 Minutes
Servings: 6

3/4 c. brown rice, cooked
3/4 c. brown Bastimi rice, cooked
1/4 c. raisins
1/4 c. fructose
1 tablespoon whole wheat flour
1/8 teaspoon pumpkin pie spice
¼ teaspoon cinnamon
¼ teaspoon nutmeg
1 cup skim milk
1 egg white, slightly beaten
1 teaspoon vanilla
Chopped walnuts (optional)

Preheat oven to 350 degrees. Combine ingredients and pour into 1 quart baking dish. Place dish in a shallow baking pan filled 1 inch deep with water. Bake 45 minutes or until center of pudding is done.

Spice Cake

Prep Time: 20 Minutes **Baking Time:** 35 Minutes
Servings: 8

1½ cup whole wheat pastry flour
2 teaspoon baking soda
1 teaspoon salt
1 teaspoon cinnamon
¼ teaspoon nutmeg
½ cup honey
6 tablespoon canola oil
1 tablespoon vinegar
½ cup water
½ cup applesauce
½ cup raisins

In medium bowl combine all dry ingredients, make a well in dry mixture. Add remaining ingredients in well. Mix well. Spoon into a 8X8 pan, sprayed with cooking spray and bake at 350° for 35 minutes. Cool in pan.

Stuffed Pears

Prep Time: 15 Minutes **Baking time:** 40 Minutes
Servings: 6

6 firm pears
¼ cup raisins
1/3 cup chopped walnuts or pecans
4 tablespoon real maple syrup
¼ teaspoon cinnamon
½ cup hot water

Preheat oven to 350°. Core pears within ¼ inch of the bottom. Combine raisins, nuts, 2 tablespoon maple syrup and cinnamon in a small bowl. Divide among pears pushing filling into cavities with a spoon handle. Place in a shallow baking dish just large enough to hold pears without crowding. Pour remaining 2 tablespoons maple syrup over pears. Pour hot water into bottom of baking dish, cover with foil and bake 40 minutes or until pears are tender when pierced with a fork. Baste pears several times during baking.

Sweet Potato Soufflé

Prep Time: 20 Minutes **Baking Time:** 70 Minutes
Servings: 6

5 fresh sweet potatoes
½ cup honey
3 tablespoon Benecol
2 egg whites
¼ teaspoon cinnamon
½ teaspoon vanilla
½ cup skim milk
½ cup chopped pecans
¼ cup molasses

Cook fresh sweet potatoes until tender—then puree. Add remaining ingredients except pecans and molasses. Bake in a casserole dish at 350° for 1 hour. Top with chopped pecans and molasses last 10 minutes of baking time.

Index

Alcohol 10, 11, 12, 28
Allspice 27
Almonds 8
Amazing Whole Wheat Bread 116, 117
Anaheim chili peppers 25
Antioxidants 8
Appetizers 32
Apple Cake 247, 249
Apple Chicken 142, 143
Apple Oatmeal Muffins 116, 130
Applesauce Loaf 247, 251
Applesauce Muffins 116, 131
Applesauce Oatmeal Cookies 247, 252

Baked Apples 247, 253
Baked Beans 197, 198
Balsamic Vinegar 27
Banana Nut Bread 116, 120
Banana Oatmeal Crispies 247, 255
Barbecue Chicken 142, 144
Barley Malt 13
Bay Leaf 26
Bean and Buffalo/Turkey Quesadilla 32, 34
Beans 18
Beef 17, 28
Bell Peppers 24
Black Bean Dip 32, 35
Black Bean Soup 52, 54
Black beans 15
Blackberry Crisps 247, 256
Blackened Halibut 142, 145
Blood 16

Blueberry Muffins 116, 132
Blueberry Streusel Muffins 247, 257
Body organs 16
Bones 16
Bran 21
Bran Muffins 116, 133
Breads 116
Broccoli Pecan Salad 71, 74
Broccoli Salad 71, 75
Brown Beans (traditional southern dish) 197, 201
Brownies 247, 258
Buffalo 17
Buffalo Chicken Tenders 32, 36
Buffalo Stew 52, 56
Buffalo/Turkey Barley Soup 52, 55

Caesar Salad 71, 76
Calcium 8, 9
Calories 2
Cancer 8
Canola Oil 22
Carbohydrate 4, 10, 12, 14
Carrot Cake 247, 260
Carrot Muffins 116, 134
Cashew Chicken Stir Fry 142, 148
Cayenne Peppers 25
Cherry Cobbler 247, 261
Chicken 17
Chicken Apple Salad 71, 78
Chicken Cabbage Salad 71, 79
Chicken Enchiladas 142, 149
Chicken Fajita Salad 71, 80

Chicken Fajitas 142, 150
Chicken Macadamia Salad 71, 81
Chicken Spaghetti 142, 151
Chicken Stew 52, 57
Chicken Vegetable and Whole Wheat Noodle Soup 52, 58
Chicken Vegetable Quesadillas 32, 37
Chili 52, 59
Chili Corn 197, 204
Chinese Coleslaw 71, 82
Chives 26
Cholesterol viii, 5, 6, 7, 17, 18, 22
Cider Vinegar 27
Cinnamon 27
Cinnamon Raisin Nut Bread 116, 117
Cinnamon Rolls 116, 121
Citrus Pomegranate Bread 116, 118
Cloves 27
Coconuts 8
Coleslaw 71, 84
Complex carbohydrates 4, 13
Copper 9
Coriander or Cilantro 26
Corn Bread 116, 123
Cornmeal 21
Crab Enchiladas 142, 153
Cranberry Muffins 116, 135
Creamy Coleslaw 71, 85
Creamy Vegetable Dip 32, 38
Crispy Baked Chicken 142, 154
Cumin 26
Curry Vegetable Dip 32, 39

Dairy Products 18, 28
Desserts 247
Dietary fiber 9
Dijon Salad Dressing 71, 109
Dill 26
Dry beans 14

Eggs 17, 24
Elk 17
Energy 1, 3, 4, 8, 9, 14
Essential amino acids 16
Essential Fatty Acids 7
Evaporated Cane Juice 13, 23

Fat 5, 17, 22
Favorite Fruit Muffins 116, 136
Fiber 8, 9, 14
Fish 17
Folic acid 9
Food 1
French Onion Soup 52, 60
French Toast 116, 138
Fresh Basil Vegetable Soup 52, 61
Fresh Fruit Pizza 247, 269
Fresh Salsa 32, 40
Fruit 15
Fruit Salsa 32, 41
Fruit Zest 28

Garlic 26
Garlic Broccoli 197, 211
Garlic Croutons 71, 77
Garlic Whole Wheat Pita Chips 32, 42
Ginger 27
Ginger Almond Chicken Stir Fry 142, 161
Ginger Bread 116, 124
Gingersnaps 247, 272
Glucose 10
Grains and Flours 21
Grandma's Lemon Grilled Chicken 142, 162
Granola 116, 139
Green Beans and Almonds 197, 212
Grilled Cajun Fish 142, 163
Grilled Chicken Quesadillas 32, 44

Grilled Corn on The Cob 197, 213
Ground turkey 17
Guacamole 32, 43

Habanero Peppers 25
Hamburger Buns 116, 125
Health 1
Healthy 1
Healthy Fat 7, 17
Heart attacks 8
Herb Mushrooms 197, 215
Herbed Chicken 142, 164
Hermits 247, 274
High blood pressure 8
High Fructose Corn Syrup 10, 28
Honey 13, 23
Honey Baked Chicken 142, 167
Hot and Sour Soup 52, 62
Hot Chicken Lettuce Salad 71, 91
Hungry 3
Hydrogenated 6
Hydrogenated fats 6
Hydrogenated or Partially Hydrogenated Fats 28

Immune system 16
Insoluble fiber 14
Insulin 10
Italian Bean Sauté 197, 217
Italian Carrots 197, 218
Italian Chicken 142, 168
Italian Vegetable Soup 52, 63

Jalapeno Cornbread 116, 126
Jalapenos 25
Juices 10, 11, 12, 28

Kick It Up A Notch Fish 142, 169, 197

Lasagna 142, 170
Legumes 18
Lemon Broccoli Pasta 197, 219
Lemon Chicken Salad 71, 92
Lemon Curry Dip 32, 45
Lemon Pepper Halibut 142, 171
Lemon Streusel 247, 276
Lentils 14
Linolenic Acid 7

Macadamia nuts 9
Magnesium 8, 9
Main Course 142
Maple Syrup 23
Margarine 22
Marinara Sauce 142, 173
Marinated Chicken Breasts 142, 172
Marinated Salmon 142, 174
Meatloaf 142, 175
Meats 17
Mexican Plate 142, 177
Mexican Turkey Burger 142, 178
Min 25
Molasses 13, 23
Molasses Rolls 116, 127
Monounsaturated fat 8
Monounsaturated fats 5, 9
Monounsaturated fatty acids 9
Muscles 16
Mushroom Tarragon Fish 142, 179
Mustard 26

Nutmeg 27
Nuts 8

Oatmeal Cookies 247, 279
Oats 21
Obesity 9

Old Fashion Tomato Soup 52, 64
Olive Oils 22
Omega-3 fatty acids 7
Omega-6 7
Onions 28
Orange Rolls 116, 122
Oregano 25
Oriental Broccoli 197, 221
Oriental Chicken Tenders 142, 181
Oven Fried Fish 142, 182
Oven Fried Zucchini 197, 222

Palm oils 8
Pancakes 116, 140
Parsley 26
Partially hydrogenated 6
Peach Berry Superb 247, 282
Peach Cobbler 281
Peanut Salad 71, 94
Peanuts 9, 16
Pecan Delights 247, 283
Pecans 8
Pepper 24, 26
Perspective on Carbohydrates 10
Perspective on Eating 1
Perspective on Fats 5
Perspective on Fiber 14
Perspective on Proteins 16
Phosphorus 9
Polyunsaturated fats 7
Popcorn Flour 21
Poppy seeds 27
Pork 17, 28
Portions 3
Potassium 9
Potatoes 10, 11, 28
Poultry 17
Protein 8, 16, 17, 18
Pumpkin Bread 116, 128

Real maple syrup 13
Red Wine Vinegar 28
Relleno Peppers 24
Rice Flour 21
Roasted Bell Peppers 197, 223
Roasted Sweet Potatoes 197, 226
Rosemary 25

Sage 25
Salad Dressing 22
Salads 71
Salmon 17
Salmon Balls 32, 46
Salmon Patties 142, 184
Saturated fat viii, 6, 17, 18
Sautéed Spinach 197, 227
Sautéed Spinach and Mushroom 197, 228
Sautéed Squash 197, 229
Savory 25
Savory Asparagus 197, 231
Savory Garlic Bread 116, 118
Selenium 8
Serrano Peppers 25
Serving 3
Shell fish 17
Sherry Vinegar 28
Silent offenders ix
    High fructose corn syrup ix
    Hydrogenated oils ix
    Potatoes ix
    Saturated fats ix
    White flour ix
    White rice ix
    White sugar ix
silent offenders ix
Simple carbohydrate 4
Simple carbohydrates 10
Soft Chicken Tacos 142, 186

Soluble fiber 14
Sorghum Syrup 24
Soups 52
Southwest Chicken 142, 187
Southwest Chicken Salad 71, 96
Southwest Vegetable or Corn Chip Dip 32, 47
Spaghetti Sauce 142, 188
Spice Cake 247, 285
Spices 25
Spicy Chicken Breasts 142, 189
Spicy Oven Fried Chicken 142, 190
Spicy Zucchini 197, 236
Spinach Artichoke Dip 32, 48
Spinach Red Onion Salad 71, 99
Spinach Salad 71, 100
Split Pea Soup 52, 65
Stevia 13
Stroke 8
Stuffed Bell Peppers 142, 191
Stuffed Mushrooms 32, 49
Sugar 10, 11
Sweet Pepper Relish 197, 238
Sweet peppers 24
Sweet Potato Salad 71, 102
Sweeteners 23
Szechwan Buffalo Stir Fry 142, 192

Taco Soup 52, 67
Tarragon 26
Teriyaki Halibut 142, 193
Thai Hot Peppers 25
Thyme 25
Tomato and Basil Stuffed Mushrooms 32, 50
Tomato Tuna Salad 71, 104
Trans Fats 6
Trans-fatty acids 7

Turkey 17
Turkey and Broccoli Lasagna 142, 195
Turkey Vegetable Soup 52, 69
Turmeric 26

Vanilla 27
Vegetable protein 16
Vegetable Soup 52, 70
Vegetable Stir Fry 197, 242
Vegetable Wrap 197, 244
Vegetables 3, 4, 12, 14, 15, 25, 197
Vegetarians 18
Vinegar 27
Vitamin E 8, 9

Waffles 116, 141
Walnuts 9
Wheat Bra 21
Wheat Bran 21
Wheat Germ 21
Wheat Germ Muffins 116, 137
White Flour 28
White flour 10, 11
White Rice 28
White rice 10, 11, 12
White Rice Vinegar 28
White Sugar 28
Whole grain 13
Whole grain pasta 13
Whole Wheat Flour 22
Whole Wheat Tortilla Chips 32, 51
Whole-grain foods 14

Zinc 8
Zucchini Bread 116, 129
5 Bean Soup 52, 53
7 Layer Mexican Dip 32, 33

978-0-595-39745-7
0-595-39745-X

Manufactured by Amazon.ca
Acheson, AB